Praise for

"Mary-Grace Fahrun has done it again. From the strong yet kind voice of *Italian Folk Magic* comes heartfelt stories meant to empower and uplift. Mary-Grace's journey will help you see the structure inherent in her system and embolden you to create your own. After all, one of the few things in this life that we truly own are the memories that shape who we are. Dive into *Living Folk Magic*, and remember who you are."
—Amy Blackthorn, author of *Blackthorn's Botanical Shadow Work*

"True to the Craft, folk witch Mary-Grace Fahrun brings us a down-to-earth, approachable, and most of all, doable guide, in her book *Living Folk Magic*. 'Living' resonates as a double-entendre throughout this book. Fahrun presents vibrant, innovative, and traditional folk practices brimming with age-old wisdom. Through her stories and guidance, curious practitioners learn to live by the folk magic of their ancestors, with respect for neighboring traditions, thereby keeping folk magic alive."
—Priestess Stephanie Rose Bird, artist, and author of numerous magical books including *Motherland Herbal, African American Magick, and Sticks, Stones, Roots and Bones*

"*Living Folk Magic* is a lantern of ancestral wisdom, guiding us back to the everyday enchantment that has always been ours. With cleansing, blessing, protection, and defense as her four steadfast pillars, Mary-Grace Fahrun shows us how to weave these timeless practices into our kitchens, homes, and hearts. Her words feel like a blessing themselves—practical, heartfelt, and brimming with the magic of real life."
—Laura Davila, author of *Mexican Magic* and *Mexican Sorcery*

"*Living Folk Magic* is about just that—living everyday life soulfully and with an intention that is at once magical and practical. Mary-Grace Fahrun teaches us that simple, heartfelt rituals often have a meaningful impact on our lives; that we are never separate from the spiritual wisdom of our ancestors; and that the world around us is thrumming with enchantment, wonder, and sacred mystery. From practicing divination and protection to communicating effectively with spirits, *Living Folk Magic* is not just a book; it's an experience—and one that we would all do well to have."
—Antonio Pagliarulo, author of *The Evil Eye* and *Queer Saints*

LIVING FOLK MAGIC

Crafting Your Own Magical Life

LIVING FOLK MAGIC

Crafting Your Own Magical Life

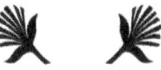

MARY-GRACE FAHRUN

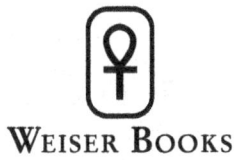

WEISER BOOKS

This edition first published in 2025 by Weiser Books, an imprint of

Red Wheel/Weiser, LLC
With offices at:
65 Parker Street, Suite 7
Newburyport, MA 01950
www.redwheelweiser.com

Copyright © 2025 by Mary-Grace Fahrun
All rights reserved. No part of this publication may be reproduced or transmitted in any form or by any means, electronic or mechanical, including photocopying, recording, or by any information storage and retrieval system, nor used in any manner for purposes of training artificial intelligence (AI) technologies to generate text or imagery, including technologies that are capable of generating works in the same style or genre, without permission in writing from Red Wheel/Weiser, LLC. Reviewers may quote brief passages.

ISBN: 978-1-57863-887-1
Library of Congress Cataloging-in-Publication Data
Names: Fahrun, Mary-Grace, 1968- author
Title: Living folk magic : crafting your own magical life / Mary-Grace Fahrun.
Description: Newburyport, MA : Weiser Books, [2025] | Summary: "Folk magic is more than casting a spell or creating a ritual. It is a way of life, a way of living, a way of perceiving the world and all within it. This book emphasizes that folk magic is not a dead thing of the past but something alive, vital, and modern, and it explores how to build an entire folk magic practice. The goal is to help readers understand folk magic so that they can actually live it and make it fulfilling and successful"-- Provided by publisher.
Identifiers: LCCN 2025025737 | ISBN 9781578638871 trade paperback | ISBN 9781578638871 ebook
Subjects: LCSH: Magic | Folklore | Spiritual life | BISAC: BODY, MIND & SPIRIT / Magick Studies | BODY, MIND & SPIRIT / Witchcraft (see also RELIGION / Wicca)
Classification: LCC BF1621 .F34 2025 | DDC 133.4/3--dc23/eng/20250821
LC record available at https://lccn.loc.gov/20

Cover design by Sky Peck Design
Interior by Steve Amarillo / Urban Design LLC
Typeset in Adobe Mrs Eaves and Mighty Script

Printed in the United States of America
IBI
10 9 8 7 6 5 4 3 2 1

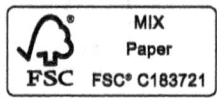

In loving memory of Donna Aquino and Teresa Giosia—this book is dedicated to you.

My dear friend and mentor, Donna Aquino—a true sister in the craft. You embodied kindness and fairness, and you taught me the sacred difference between being kind and being nice. Your wisdom, strength, and spirit live on in all you touched.

My dear soul sister, Teresa Giosia—Sisters in the craft from the very beginning, walking this path side by side. You were a force of nature—full of light, laughter, and a childlike wonder that never dimmed. Wherever you went, you brought sunshine. I carry your light and love with me always.

This book contains advice and information relating to herbs and is not meant to diagnose, treat, or prescribe. It should be used to supplement, not replace, the advice of your physician or other trained healthcare practitioner. Some herbs are poisonous and should be used with extreme care. If you know or suspect you have a medical condition, if you are experiencing physical symptoms, or if you feel unwell, seek your physician's advice before embarking on any medical program or treatment. Readers using the information in this book do so entirely at their own risk, and the author and publisher accept no liability if adverse effects are caused.

Table of Contents

Introduction	I
Chapter 1: The Four Pillars	II
Chapter 2: Qualities, Skills, and Responsibilities of the Folk Witch	25
Chapter 3: Diasporic Folk Magic: History, Spells, and Tools	55
Chapter 4: Enchanted World: Animism in Folk Magic	91
Chapter 5: Building Sacred Bonds: Cultivating Relationships with Spirits	99
Chapter 6: Dreams, Trance, Spirit Flight, and Time Travel in Folk Magic	119
Chapter 7: A Guide to Safe and Discreet Practice	139
Chapter 8: Common Folk Magic Spells from Around the World	159
Chapter 9: Conclusion	183
Chapter 10: Unearthing the Roots: A Practical Guide to Finding Information	197
Acknowledgments	207

Introduction

Folk magic exists in every culture and has been practiced since the dawn of time. Folk magic is a practice consisting of cultural customs, folklore, magic, superstitions, and religious beliefs. It is a way for humans to interact with and understand both the physical and nonphysical world around them. It involves recognizing the presence of both seen and unseen, living and nonliving entities. Folk magic often arises from necessity, as practitioners turn to it when all other practical options have failed. While the rituals and practices of folk magic aim to communicate with spirits or divine forces, they are usually combined with practical efforts to achieve a desired outcome. I view spell work and rituals as an external expression of prayer, where symbolic actions and words set the stage for spiritual or divine intervention.

These practices focus on solving everyday problems, such as healing, ensuring a good harvest, finding lost items, attracting love or good fortune, and protecting against misfortune or evil spirits. As mentioned, folk magic is deeply rooted in cultural traditions, and it blends superstition and religion. The practices vary based on culture and belief system.

Anyone familiar with Roman Catholicism will recognize its influence in my practice, especially in the presence of Catholic iconography, some of the spirits I invoke, and the items I use. My folk magic is supported by what I have come to call the "four pillars of folk magic." Much like the four legs of a table or the four walls of a room, these pillars are the foundation of my practice. They serve to provide stability, structure, and protection:

Cleansing: to remove negative energy

Blessing: to imbue with love

Protection: to charge with energy that repels evil

Defense: to combat evil

These four pillars are certainly applicable to any cultural and spiritual practice. When I bless an object, for example, I commonly use holy water and will recite an incantation over the object. To outsiders, this blessing looks like Catholicism. To Catholics raised aware of these practices but not practicing them, it may be viewed as superstition. To non-Catholic Christians, it is viewed as witchcraft or, at the very least, blasphemous. It is not possible to extricate the Catholic components from Italian folk magic without losing a main source of power. I know this firsthand because I have experimented over the years leaving out the Catholic components. Although it was fine, my magic was significantly underpowered, and when the proverbial poop hit the ventilator, I quickly reinserted the Catholic components, and the boost in power was instantaneous. I will discuss why I think this is. Animism is also inextricably woven into this magical tapestry. Upon close inspection of my ancestors' cultural customs, beliefs, and superstitions, animism is the dominant spiritual belief. It is this dominant belief in animism that links the sacred and the profane. My favorite example that illustrates this is when my ancestors would say, "Garlic is Saint Michael." Garlic has a spirit. It is both garlic and Michael the Archangel. A mere clove of garlic holds the power of and *is* Michael the Archangel.

I want to go beyond the surface level of folk magic and get down to the bones of it—what we are doing when we call upon a spirit to help us to find lost objects, recite an incantation to remove the evil eye, or wear a talisman for potency. I wish to discuss these common practices further and to provide context—explain why we do them and hypothesize what I think makes them work. Because they do work. You don't even have to be Catholic for Saint Anthony to help you find what you have lost. You don't have to believe in the evil eye for the cure to clear a headache you have had for three weeks just fifteen minutes after the ritual was performed to remove it.

More importantly, I want to discuss in earnest the animism at the core of folk magic because it is such an integral part of my belief system and reality. The folk witch is one who dances with the saints and the sinners, the living and the nonliving, and their power relies on and is commensurate with their ability to forge strong relationships with their spirits. When I refer to the spirits, this includes but is not limited to guardian angels, saints, ancestors, and spirit guides in all forms such as animal, plant, and mineral, and from all realms. These relationships take courage, time, discernment, and finesse. We need to be comfortable with not knowing anything for sure. Furthermore, relationships between the folk witch and the spirits require a give-and-take from both the witch and the spirits. Trust and loyalty are earned, be it by the living or the nonliving. But once trust and loyalty are established, bonds beyond space and time are formed. Lastly, ours is a solitary path, but we do not work alone.

Cursed and Called: My Entry into Folk Witchcraft

Before I get down to the business of exploring how to build an entire folk magic practice, I think it would be helpful if I told you the story of how I came to this practice.

I was born into a culture and to a family where religion and superstition seemed to be one and the same. *Healer fortune-tellers* (what we would call a *folk witch* today, but they never identified as such) were respected members of our community and consulted regularly. Our beloved dead continued to participate and assist us in our daily lives. We maintained open dialogue with them by speaking to them. They responded by appearing in our dreams and sending us signs. We kept their memory alive for those who never got to meet them through the retelling of their stories and the maintaining of traditions they passed down to us. Even religious figures such as God, Jesus, the Blessed Virgin, saints, and angels were spoken about and experienced as though they were members of our family. The healer fortune-tellers were revered; alternatively, those who were known to be spellcasters were feared. The threat of the evil eye, misfortune, curses, and malefic spirits were believed to be always present, and we did some things to protect ourselves that were, for lack of a better word, witchy. However, this behavior is not unique to my culture. In every culture, a subset of the population leans more into cultural spiritual beliefs and practices, superstitions, and witchcraft. I also feel we know pretty early on if we belong to that subset of the population. We experience something that puts us directly in touch with the supernatural that opens our eyes and challenges all our beliefs.

In the summer of 1985, I had my first tarot reading. I found a listing for a psychic who advertised in our daily newspaper. I phoned the number on the listing and booked my appointment for the following afternoon.

I could hardly contain my excitement on the bus ride to my appointment in Little Italy. I found the tiny old house and rang the doorbell. I was let in and asked to wait by the entrance. I was invited into the tiny room to the right of the front door. There were stark white plaster walls, moist with humidity, with Catholic saints iconography cut from old calendars affixed to the wall with thumbtacks. A candle, encased in a tall red glass jar, was burning. There was a tiny foldout table and two foldout chairs. There were cards on the table, but not the Neapolitan or the poker playing cards I read. These were larger in size, well worn and coffee stained. The pattern on the backs of the cards was a faded blue plaid. There was the scent of church incense in the air.

The psychic appeared to be in her twenties. She was tall, thin, pale, with thick, shiny raven hair down to her waist that she deftly gathered into an updo as I entered the room. She had huge, round, almost black eyes framed by the thickest, darkest eyelashes I'd ever seen. It was summer, and it was hot and humid in her house. She wore a white tank top and a colorful flowy skirt. She introduced herself and said she was the descendant of "a long line of Sicilian seers."

She invited me to sit in a chair facing her, not at the table with the cards. We sat facing each other and close enough for our knees to touch. She gripped my hands and muttered what sounded like a prayer in Arabic or Sicilian, or both. She pressed her forehead to mine. Then she strengthened her grip on my hands, threw her head back, and snapped her head forward; all the while her almost-black eyes gazed deeply into mine. I lost all sensation of my body and spatial awareness.

She told me things about people close to me that she could not possibly know. She told me of my grief, and the pain and rage I kept contained, and the secrets I kept that I had not told a soul. She described people I hadn't met yet—including physical descriptions and nationalities—but whom I did end up meeting just a few months later. She described a future relationship with "an intelligent and charismatic person" wrought with very specific personal problems. This also came to pass. "You have to help them," she said to me with urgency.

She told me I would arrive at a crossroads regarding my career. Neither choice was in my awareness at the time. She said I would choose the hard road. I scoffed a little. This too came to pass and played out exactly like she described. It was damn hard. She told me things I kept buried deep, deep inside myself, things I hadn't been able to tell myself but knew to be true.

She released her grip on my hands, and I felt myself fall back into my body and once again became aware of the uncomfortable chair I was sitting in. She then reached for her cards. I asked about them because I had never seen anything like them. She told me they were tarot cards. The first card she drew was a woman wearing a blindfold surrounded by eight swords. The second card was The Devil. "You are cursed," she said. It sounded like a question she was asking herself. Then she straightened herself up and repeated, only this time with more authority: "Someone put a curse on you. It will cost $1,000 in cash to remove it." She proceeded to give me instructions on what I needed to do—from taking a bath to praying a novena (consisting of special prayers on nine successive days).

I stopped her right there. "I don't have $1,000."

"You can borrow it," she urged.

"Really? *Who* in that cast of characters you just described from my life is going to lend me $1,000 for me to pay you to remove a curse?"

She continued to say that she knew I could find the money.

"No, I cannot."

"What are you going to do?" she inquired. "You can't remain like this!"

I didn't answer her. I pulled the cash out of my wallet and placed my $30 for the reading on the table as she had instructed me to do when I first arrived, and I left. I walked down to the Catholic church at the end of the street. It was late afternoon; it was blazing hot on the church steps. The air was filled with the scent of stone and old wood baking in the hot July sun. I gripped the scorching hot iron door handle. It was locked. I pushed on the door. It didn't open. I collapsed under the oppressive heat and lit a cigarette. Despondent. Godless. Cursed.

The long bus ride home gave me time to think. I remembered that my great aunt had taught me just a few summers ago how to defend myself magically against curses. I couldn't quite remember what to do other than I would have to know who had cursed me and how it may have been done. I couldn't understand why someone would have cursed me. How would I even begin to find out who and how they did it? If my great aunt were still alive, she would know how to help me.

Over the next year, I watched my life unfold before me exactly as the psychic had predicted, down to every minute detail. The reading was so spookily accurate that I began to question whether she had made it all happen. Since we were kids, my friends and I had always exchanged card readings. I asked them to read for me on numerous occasions that year. Neither of them ever said anything about a curse in my cards, but that did not console me. Dread was my constant companion, and the thought that I was cursed added an undercurrent of hopelessness. I began to spend hours and hours for days on end at our public library reading anything I could find on curses and witchcraft, in both English and French. I filled a three-ring binder with Xerox copies of portions of books and copious notes on loose-leaf paper. When I didn't have money for Xerox copies, I wrote down my notes by hand and drew the images from the books. My binder of notes and sketches, a copy of *Le Arti Magiche* (*The Magical Arts*) by Hermes Edizioni purchased at the Italian bookstore, and my Rider-Waite tarot cards lived in my backpack. I never left home without it.

One day, when everyone was out, I grabbed a shallow white bowl, filled it with water, and poured three drops of olive oil onto the water to check myself for *malocchio* (the Italian name for the evil eye). For the last three days, I had suffered a headache. My thought process was that if the test was positive, I could attempt to remove the evil eye, and in the process the curse would also be removed.

The drops of olive oil landed in the water and vanished. "That's not good," I thought to myself. Now what? I knew the prayer and the incantation to cure the evil eye, but the cure consisted of Catholic prayers. I couldn't do it. It's not that I didn't try. Reciting prayers felt unnatural and stilted. It had been eight years since my last confession and at least seven years since I left the Church. I attempted the cure to dispel the evil eye, skipping over all the Catholic parts of the prayer and incantation. There wasn't much left to recite. I did it anyway.

The headache seemed to abate a little. Not completely. I heard someone coming home. I quickly washed and put everything away and returned to my room. I opened my newly acquired copy of *Le Arti Magiche* to search for any information that could assist me in removing this curse. There was none. There was, however, a lot of information on how to curse, and all those curses required something belonging to the person being cursed and some body part belonging to an animal. Horrified, I slammed the book shut and threw it in my backpack. I flipped through my binder instead. Maybe I could reverse engineer a cure from the instructions on how to curse—but minus harming any animals. I had no idea where to start, and honestly, by this point, even the information I had gathered in my binder was starting to creep me out.

The headache, now low-grade but ever present, persisted for weeks—joined by new symptoms of low-grade nausea, loss of appetite, and a persistent feeling of dread of impending doom. When I pulled tarot cards for myself, they were all what my friends and I called the "black" cards—The Devil, The Tower, Nine of Swords, Ten of Swords, Five of Pentacles—literally, the cards in my deck of Rider-Waite tarot that were mainly black in color. I was new to tarot, and these cards filled me with dread and foreboding. I finally confided to my friend whose family was also from Naples. I told him about the reading I'd had over a year ago and that the psychic said I was cursed. I told him she wanted $1,000 to remove the curse.

"What did you do?" he asked.

"Nothing," I replied and added, "It's probably a scam."

He looked at me and, in all seriousness, asked, "What if it's true?" He grabbed me by my hand and said, "Come on," and before I could ask where he was taking me, he said, "I'm taking you to Grandma's house."

When we arrived, my friend's grandma greeted us with open arms and offered us something to eat. My friend whispered something in her ear, and she looked at me and said, "Oh, my God!" She had me pick a walnut from a bowl and place it on the table. She smashed the walnut open with the palm of her open hand. The walnut meat inside the shell was moldy and shriveled. She gasped and got a bowl from her kitchen cupboard, filled it with water, and poured three drops of olive oil into the bowl of water to confirm what she suspected from the shriveled walnut—that the evil eye was present. The three drops of oil disappeared in the water. Oil and water don't mix. However, when one is checking for the evil eye, if the oil disappears in the water, it confirms the subject (in this case, me) is afflicted. My friend joined his grandma as she proceeded to recite the incantation to dispel the evil eye.

With each repetition of the incantation, I ran to the toilet and filled it with vomit, although my stomach was empty, as I had not eaten for days. Finally, the retching stopped, and I collapsed on the floor, exhausted and soaked in sweat. My friend picked me up and helped me to the sofa. In the meantime, my friend's grandma checked me with the olive oil and water again, and she rejoiced, clapping her hands and singing that all was well.

I opened my eyes and for a moment forgot where I was. My friend's grandma said, "My God, child, where have you been?"

"Did I have a curse?" I asked.

She exclaimed, "No! You had nothing but a *touch* of the evil eye. Most likely inflicted by the same amateur witch you went to see to have your cards read."

I looked at my friend, and he smiled apologetically and said, "I'm sorry. I had to tell her."

Grandma fed us and sent us on our way. As we were leaving, I thanked, hugged, and kissed her, and she pressed a prayer card of Saint Michael the Archangel in my hand saying, "He will always be with you now." After stepping out into the sunshine, I couldn't stop marveling to my friend how the world was amazingly bright and colorful. I didn't realize I was under a black cloud until it was lifted.

A decade later, my friend's grandma would confess to me that it was, in fact, a curse and that "the witch that read your cards was no amateur." She explained that to have acknowledged the full force of both in that precarious moment would feed it. Diminishing the curse by calling it a "a *touch* of the evil eye by an amateur" starved it and rendered its removal more easily attainable.

One would think that having had this experience would have made me fearful and run in the other direction from witchcraft. Instead, it made witchcraft even more attractive to me. Consumed with the need to understand the workings of the unseen world, I jumped in feet first and never looked back. This is where my life in folk magic began.

Chapter 1

The Four Pillars

The number one question posed to me over the course of the last twenty-five years, and especially in the last five years, is "What does your folk magic practice look like? Do you practice exactly as your ancestors did?"

The short answer is yes because Italian folk magic makes up the bones of my practice, whether I want it to be or not. The long answer is far more nuanced. The flesh of my practice is composed of my lived experience informed by my trial (and much error or, rather, lack of success) and the modifications that were born of my necessity, accessibility, availability, the spirits of the land upon which I live, and the cross-pollination that naturally occurs through interaction with other practitioners of various cultures and traditions.

Nothing in this book is presented as absolute fact, but I can promise that everything is true to my personal experience with folk magic. While I'm not an anthropologist, I've worked in health care for my entire adult life. As a trained observer, I am always assessing and analyzing, whether I'm awake or asleep. My approach is influenced by the scientific method and the nursing process, which help me observe, gather information, analyze, predict outcomes, experiment, solve problems, and innovate. From my healthcare experience, I understand how helpful routines and structures are for evaluating results and spotting patterns or issues. In this chapter, I will share the structure I use in my practice, which is rooted in ancestral folk magic but adapted to modern life.

I don't intend to impose my framework on anyone. My goal is simply to share my magical perspective and processes in the hope of inspiring both beginners and experienced practitioners alike. My magico-spiritual practices are flexible, and this framework is what gives them structure.

Just as my ancestors did not have a name for their magico-spiritual practices, neither do I, if I am honest. I mean, for expediency in communication with other practitioners, I will use terms such as *folk magic practitioner* and *folk witch* interchangeably, but those terms don't really capture the whole depth and breadth of this thing that really has no name.

If my ancestors were pressed, they would say, "These are the things we do," and there were phrases they would use to hint at their degree of involvement in "the things we do." These people who believed in folk magic and folk witchery but were devout Catholics who would never call themselves folk magic or folk healing practitioners, but didn't completely discount the customs and practices, would describe themselves on one end of the spectrum as "a little superstitious." This expression captures most of my family and community, who would say: "It's not real, but I believe."

At the complete other end of the spectrum were the metaphysicians and occultists, and they identified themselves with the statement: "I am VERY superstitious." This is code for the people who were, by our modern definitions, full-on practicing witches and/or shamans. Between "a little superstitious" and "VERY superstitious" is a whole spectrum of degrees of involvement.

Forty years ago, when I was a teen attracted to the occult, I would have described myself as curious and a little superstitious. If I were to use the phraseology of my ancestors to describe myself today . . . well, let's just say that I am very superstitious, and these are the things I do.

My Four Pillars of Folk Magic

A few years ago, I realized that my magical practice has a core structure, composed of fundamental actions that are consistently present in my life. In my mind's eye, I envision these actions as what I call "the four pillars." The four pillars of my practice are cleansing, blessing, protection, and defense. My magical practice isn't something separate from me or confined to a set time, like every Monday at 7:00 p.m. Instead, these four pillars are woven into every aspect of my life. The depth of my engagement with them shifts depending on my family and work responsibilities, my mood, my state of mind and body, and, most importantly, my needs. By needs, I mean that when I'm facing any challenge—whether mundane or spiritual—my connection with the four pillars becomes more intentional and focused. When life is flowing smoothly, my engagement with the pillars is more subtle. I often compare it to a computer's operating system: The foundation is always there, offering stability and boundaries, even when it's not in the forefront. At this point in my life, these actions are so deeply ingrained in my routine that they've become second nature. To write about them, I had to reflect on my daily practices and carefully identify what I now recognize as the four pillars.

Cleansing

The first pillar is cleansing. Cleansing in this context is extremely broad and, by both my observation and experience, the most essential practice. The simple act of cleansing can instantly transform a person, place, or situation. In my family and community, everything begins and ends with cleansing. The act is very simple; the effects are all encompassing. Cleansing begins with the physical actions of cleaning, tidying up one's person and surroundings and washing. Cleansing goes deeper, however. With cleansing, one is not only removing dirt and germs, via washing, but one is also in a spiritual sense cleansing the person and their surroundings of unfavorable energy and evil spirits. Cleaning physically loosens and removes dirt. Cleansing spiritually loosens and removes energetic accumulation. I view cleansing as spiritually sanitizing the space once it is clean. Cleansing can be done with spoken words, fire (such as lighting a candle, for instance), smoke (fumigating with herbs or incense), salt (sprinkling it on surfaces and then sweeping it away and out of the home), and water (sprinkling holy water).

In my youth, it annoyed me to no end when the elders of my community gave the same advice for absolutely every human condition:

In a bad mood? Wash your face.

Feeling sad? Take a bath.

Feeling agitated? Take a bath.

Feeling frustrated? Clean the house.

Feeling listless? Clean the house.

Feeling angry? Clean the house.

Feeling argumentative or spoiling for a fight? Keep your mouth shut and—you guessed it—clean the house.

You see, the elders believed that evil spirits—or, alternatively, people's evil intentions—were whirling around us at such times, sowing seeds of indolence and discord, and that cleaning the house and washing the body removed these seeds and sent the evil spirits packing.

Sounds crazy right? I thought so too. But you know what? It always worked. I freely admit that, even as a cynical teenager, I always experienced and observed that the environment felt better. I felt better. This advice worked then and it still works now. Try it and see for yourself.

In actual practice, cleaning is an element of cleansing, and both are carried out simultaneously, incorporating all earthly elements of air, fire, water, and earth. From cleansing a space such as a room, a vehicle, the garden, to cleansing an object such as a rock or tabletop prior to use in ritual, cleansing can be carried out with any or all four elements, whatever is safe and appropriate.

To give a concrete example, before I begin a project, I clear my desk or whichever surface I will be working on. I air out the space by opening a window, wipe down the surface with a damp cloth, and light a candle. I do this every time. This act of cleansing is so automatic that I don't even think about it.

Blessing

The next pillar is blessing. The act of blessing involves directing the energy of love, gratitude, and good wishes upon the target of the blessing. Blessing is a magical act with the purpose to produce positive outcomes, good luck, health, and prosperity.

Between you and me, don't tell anyone I told you this, but I can be a bit of a complainer. Even when life is good, I can find something that isn't. I blame this on my Italian DNA because, honestly, I do sound like my parents when I pick out the one thing that isn't perfect in an otherwise decent if not downright wonderful situation. Being self-aware, I make sure to catch myself before complaining, and if it's too late and the complaint slips out, I always make sure to follow up with blessings and words of gratitude for the same thing I just devalued. Why? Because the elders always said to "thank God for everything, even your problems, because it can always be worse." Okay, I know. The elders were a little pessimistic, but I cut them some slack because as I've gotten older, I see more and more that their pessimism was how they guarded themselves against jinxing an outcome. Pessimism was their version of "knock on wood." Blessing is also a ward against the malocchio (evil eye). When you're complimenting a person, it is polite to follow with "May you be blessed" to dispel any envy, conscious or unconscious, or simply not to jinx it. An example would be "I am so happy to hear your doctor gave you a clean bill of health. Thank God. Knock on wood!" The elders blessed everything.

My late aunt in Italy cursed about how tired she was, having to take her cow out to pasture every day. The job was physically demanding, and she was in her eighties. She couldn't leave her cow for fear that the cow would be attacked by predators or stolen. The cow lived in a stall adjacent to her kitchen with a cut-out window, so that her cow was safe, warm, and neither one of them was ever lonely. When I was a child, I spent a summer in Italy with my aunt. Together we would clean out the stall and fill it with fresh hay daily. She brushed her cow's coat, sang blessings to her, and gave thanks to the spirits that watched over them both. It is okay to vent our frustrations, but then we need to get over ourselves and move past them.

Blessings can be bestowed with song, as in this example of my aunt singing blessings to her cow. Blessings also can be bestowed with service and a loving touch. When preparing food, handle the food gently, lovingly, and giving thanks to the animal and plant spirits of the food you are about to prepare. If the quality of the food does not meet your expectations or the dish you prepared does not turn out the way you wanted it to, refrain from complaining and bless it. This last recommendation is a hard one for me to remember because I struggle with perfectionism and just general crankiness. My husband will gently nudge me to not let perfect be the enemy of good. This nudging prompts me to bless and give thanks instead of getting caught up in my ridiculousness.

Hate is a very strong emotion, and popular psychology posits that what we hate about others is what we hate about ourselves (or something to that effect). Engaging in a little introspection can perhaps uncover those elements you hate in yourself. This can be your call to action to work on yourself or at the very least to recognize what gets a rise out of you. On the other hand, it can just be that you see how fake or even evil that person or thing is, and your hate is justified. Here, then, the call to action is to eject the person or the thing out of your life. Bless it and send it on its way.

We can bless people, objects, and environments with our thoughts and our words. We can use items such as holy water, holy oil, salt, incense, and—my favorites—perfumed waters and cologne.

Some gestures that can be used to bless people, situations, objects, and environments are making the Christian sign of the cross, patting gently and lovingly with your open dominant hand, and the laying on of one or both hands. You should use a gesture you instantly associate with blessing. Alternatively, you can adapt or create your own gesture.

The methods of blessing are not limited to my examples and are as unique as the individual. It may feel more natural to you to use a hand gesture from your culture and/or religion. What matters is that you connect to the meaning of the gesture, and by connecting to the gesture, you will instantly transfer blessing energy with it. Find a method that feels right for you and practice it often so that it becomes second nature.

Protection

The next pillar is protection. Protection is a magical act that accompanies the physical act of keeping your person and property safe. Protection wards are a key component in all kinds of religious and magical traditions. I like to think of it as my spiritual security system. Of all four pillars, protection is the one that I prioritize maintaining no matter what. Think of it as keeping your home locked and secure whether you have had time to clean or do the laundry. Protection begins with keeping your physical body safe from physical harm—from dressing appropriately for the weather so as not to risk heat exhaustion or frostbite, for example, to looking both ways before crossing the street. Basic safety, right? Same goes for magical protection.

Protection for me consists of two components that work in tandem to form my spiritual security system. The first of the two components is detection. Energetic boundaries and wards function as a surveillance system that detects any anomalies. Wards are protection spells. They can be invisible spells and may also consist of items displayed in the home that are charged with protection magic. Sensations in my body can help me detect when something is not right. A sudden feeling of dread or impending doom, unwarranted or unprovoked anger, a sudden wave of nausea or a feeling of despair—any or all of these can be signs that my body is detecting malignant energy. The second component of protection is defense. This component consists of the capture, removal, and disposal of the spiritual invader.

Setting up wards, for me, consists of several different things. There are amulets I always have in place and rituals I carry out as part of daily life. Amulets break when they take the energetic hit on our behalf and must be replaced. Physical barriers become weakened or, in some cases, breached and must be maintained, such as freshening up the salt on our windowsills and trimming the vines of a houseplant that has taken an energetic hit. Another barrier consists of spiritual protection. At the bare minimum, I check in with my spirits to feed them with offerings I know they enjoy, and I thank them for having my back.

A consistent practice of protection work is easily incorporated in even the most hectic of lives and must be prioritized. Protection offers both security and detection, and detecting breaches of our protective barrier is key to maintaining protection. For example, I have several houseplants and an intimate relationship with their spirits. Every now and then, one of my plants will either die or wither for no mundane reason. They are watered and fed and get enough light, etc. But suddenly a plant or a part of it will show sudden abnormal signs of stress, illness, or decay (detection of a breach in the protection). In these cases, I have learned to read the reason as the plant taking an energetic hit for me or a member of my family. I give thanks to the plant's spirit and, when possible, salvage what I can from it and repot it if necessary. If it is unsalvageable, the plant is put to rest. Doing so also prompts me to beef up my spiritual protection.

Have you ever felt someone's energy or will coming up against your energetic boundaries? It may feel like a tidal wave of grief, frustration, and rage. Here is something I discovered by accident simply because I talk with my hands, like many people. While this is mostly known as an "Italian thing," honestly, I have seen people of all cultures gesture with their hands when they speak. In my long career as a health-care professional, I often met people for the first time on the worst day of their lives. Every person handles health crises differently, and sometimes these crises bring out the worst in people in the form of aggressive communication or downright aggression. When interacting with people in such scenarios, I would hold out my open hands, palms facing the person, and remain calm and empathetic. This gesture could very well be one I picked up from a family member or a completely natural reflex. But it worked to keep that energy from affecting me. A similar gesture is to hold out your dominant hand, open with your palm facing the direction of someone spreading discord or negativity. I use this a lot in countless scenarios because it is so second nature to me at this point. The purpose is pretty much to repel incoming negativity, which takes us to the next pillar, defense.

I tend to use protection and defense not interchangeably but as a team. Protection magic is proactive and preventative, designed to create a shield around a person, space, or object to keep negative influences, harm, or spiritual attacks at bay. It establishes ongoing safety before any threat arises. Defensive magic, on the other hand, is reactive, used to respond to an active threat or attack. It aims to neutralize or block harmful energies, curses, or malicious forces that are already present. While protection magic prevents harm from happening, defensive magic directly defends against harm that is actively occurring. Both forms of magic are often used together, with protection establishing a foundation and defensive magic providing a targeted response when needed.

Defense

The final pillar is defense—the active or offensive action of protection. While protection is like the moat around a castle and the drawbridge, defense is the command given to the army (or dragon) to attack.

Of the four pillars, defense is probably the one I employ the least, mainly because, as the saying goes, "an ounce of prevention is worth a pound of cure." Strong protection often eliminates the need for defensive action. However, there are times when defensive magic becomes necessary. One example is when you know someone is actively working against you—perhaps attempting to discredit or sabotage you in a way that threatens your livelihood.

As with protection magic, the first step in defense magic is to take all necessary mundane actions to safeguard yourself. Once that foundation is set, defensive magic should follow immediately. My preferred methods are the ground, salt, and the freezer—quick, accessible techniques that require no special ingredients or tools. In most cases, these are sufficient to halt an attack.

It is also wise to consult your spirit court, the team of spirits that guide and protect you, informing them that something is afoot, that you have initiated your defense, and that you request their vigilance. Ask them to "stand guard" and be prepared to act if further escalation is required. This initial level of defense creates space for the practitioner to escalate to stronger measures if needed.

How to Use the Four Pillars

The four pillars form the foundation of my magico-spiritual practice. While my practice is fluid—constantly shifting, adapting, and varying in intensity—the structure they provide remains constant. I see the four pillars as a vessel that contains my practice, much like the banks of a river guide its flow.

These pillars give me a sense of routine and stability, especially during stressful or challenging times. In moments of intense emotion or uncertainty, they become the four walls of a metaphorical room—a space where I can retreat, catch my breath, and regain my center. This is why maintaining this structure during calm and stable periods is so essential. When life inevitably throws its challenges, having established routines and boundaries provides a solid foundation. Practices that become second nature, requiring no thought or effort, are invaluable when navigating life's unpredictable twists and turns.

Additionally, and probably the most important thing is that the four pillars are portable. These practices go with us wherever we go. They are skills, and they are transferable. The four pillars are applicable anywhere and, in any circumstance, folk witches would find themselves.

Here is an example of what this looks like in real life:

> **Cleansing:** At the end of my workday, I put everything away in its place, and I physically tidy my workspace. I physically clean surfaces and take out the trash and empty the recycling. I then cleanse the space of any stagnant or discordant energy. I like to keep Florida water in a little spray bottle for this purpose. If I am working in a scent-free environment, I will clap my hands three times or ring a tiny bell. If I didn't do this at the end of my previous workday, I will do it at the start of the next workday.

Blessing: I give thanks to my space and the spirits of place and things for assisting me to do my work. When appropriate, I will make an offering. Usually, it is as simple as a misting of Florida water or whatever cologne I am using at that time. Florida water, for example, is my favorite because it is an all-rounder. I use it to quickly cleanse a space or objects, to bless, and as an offering to my spirits. Other times, if working from home, I light a candle and/or a stick of incense.

Protection: I check on my wards (both physical and energetic) to make sure they are holding strong. On the mundane level, this task is making sure that windows, doors, gates, etc., are closed and secured.

Defense: The last pillar is defense. If I feel the need for it, I will initiate defensive magic. The two most common spells are Freeze Enemy spell, a classic form of defensive magic used to halt an enemy's harmful actions, prevent gossip, or stop ongoing negative influences; and MirrorSpell, used to reflect harmful energy, psychic attacks, or curses back to their source.

The structure of the four pillars applies to every space I inhabit and everything I do. While the specific methods of cleansing, blessing, protection, and defense may vary, the core principles remain unchanged. These pillars function as an energetic barrier that constantly surrounds me—and those in my care—like a portable, invisible, electrified fence. The daily maintenance of these practices is what supplies the energy that keeps this protective barrier active and strong.

You can begin building your very own (or enhance your understanding of your existing) folk magic practice right now just by introducing the four pillars into your daily life. Giving specific examples is hard because everyone's life is so different. Please read the following with the understanding that you do not have to follow any of the actions by the letter. What matters is that you apply the principles as they are the most accessible to you.

The four pillars of folk magic can be applied to your mind and physical body. Starting and ending your day with focus sets these pillars around your mind and body:

Cleansing: Start by physically cleaning your body—bathe, wash your hair, brush your teeth, and wear clean clothes. Drink a glass of water in the morning with the intention of cleansing your body from the inside. Do the same at the end of the day or before bed.

Blessing: Show unconditional love and gratitude for the body you are in, no matter how you feel about your appearance or abilities. This might be challenging, but it's important to bless your body daily. Using nice-smelling soap, wearing comfortable clothing, and resting when you're sick or injured are simple ways to bless your body.

Protection: Protect your body from harm by dressing appropriately for the weather, washing your hands to prevent illness, and choosing foods that make you feel good. Protect yourself by setting personal boundaries and avoiding activities that harm your mental health. Ensuring your physical safety is another form of protection.

Defense: Defending yourself can mean learning a martial art, consulting a doctor when you're ill, or taking prescribed medication. Going no-contact with someone who is harmful to you is also a form of defense.

A folk magic practice begins with the foundation, and the rest is built on that foundation. Establishing the four pillars within our bodies leads to the expression of the four pillars in our environment. As within so without.

A magical life is sustained by countless small actions, each one keeping the flow of magic active—just as the continuous circulation of blood keeps the body alive. These daily practices, no matter how small, ensure that magic remains present, vibrant, and integrated into every aspect of life.

Chapter 2

Qualities, Skills, and Responsibilities of the Folk Witch

A folk witch, both historically and in the modern world, is someone who embodies a unique blend of practical wisdom, intuitive insight, and deep spiritual connection. Rooted in the traditions of their ancestors, folk witches possess an intimate knowledge of herbs, energy work, and divination, using these skills to heal, protect, and guide their communities. They are resourceful, empathetic, and deeply attuned to the natural world, viewing magic not as a relic of the past but as a living, vibrant practice that adapts to the present day. They balance their craft with a profound sense of responsibility, understanding that their work—whether in cleansing, blessing, cursing, or communicating with spirits—requires both ethical awareness and a commitment to personal growth. Through this blend of tradition and modernity, folk witches continue to nurture their craft, ensuring that it remains relevant and fulfilling in an ever-changing world.

Once I observed the routine and structure of my practice, it naturally led me to ponder the qualities, skills, and responsibilities of the practitioner within that structure. I began my journey down this path by jumping in with both feet. I did not view witchcraft as a practice separate from mundane life. I viewed it as a skill set to add to my survival toolbox. Nowadays, I view folk magic as how I live my life. In those early years, I never pondered the deeper, more meaningful or existential questions such as "What kind of practitioner do I want to be?" I just wanted to know everything and have the instant ability to cast spells to give me a sense of control over my own fate. I still think that was as good a place to start as any. So, if you are reading this book and that's where you are, my advice to you is this: Roll up your sleeves and start experimenting. Be a sponge. Gather as much information as you can on what interests you. Curiosity and a desire to learn will take you far. Be open to everything, but at the same time, cultivate discernment and use your judgment. Discernment comes from experience, ours and observing the experiences of others—in questioning what we are reading or being told, maintaining our boundaries and knowing our worth, knowing who we are and what is right for us.

I believe it is important to ask yourself, "What kind of practitioner do I want to be?" or "What does being a practicing folk magician mean to me?" For me, the answer is twofold: I want to continue along the thread of the practitioners in my family and spiritual community, honoring their traditions. At the same time, I want to weave my own unique path, with that original thread running through it. I also aspire to stay connected to those who come after me, ensuring that this thread of tradition continues.

It is never too early to begin learning how to be an elder. Simply by being alive today, we are already ancestors to those who will come after us. I believe that folk magicians are bound by a thread that connects us to those who came before us and those who will follow. To walk this path with integrity, we must cultivate certain qualities, develop specific skills, and embrace key responsibilities. This alignment with our ancestors—whether of blood, spirit, or land—helps us gain their favor, guidance, and protection. My understanding of what makes a true practitioner of folk magic has grown from observing the matriarchs and patriarchs in my family and community. They inspire me even now, long after they have left this mortal plane, and I strive to embody the wisdom and strength they carried.

If you want to be a strong folk magic practitioner, it's important that you understand the core principles of folk magic. I've always been someone who needs to take things apart to understand how they work. When I see a skill that fascinates me and aligns with my practice, I don't just want to learn it—I have to. I keep learning until it becomes second nature. For me, having a variety of skills is a form of preparedness. Learning helps reduce feelings of helplessness and fear of the unknown. It also fosters independence, and independence brings freedom—which is power. Knowing the core principles of folk magic means being able to practice effectively, no matter what tools are available. It is understanding the rules of the unseen world and how to work within them.

That doesn't mean I need to know everything. What's important is knowing what I need for my practice—and knowing it well. Every practitioner has different strengths. Some are skilled in astrology, some in herbalism, and others in working with spirits or deities. There are many paths within folk magic, and no one person has to master them all. The best part of folk magic is that learning never stops. Whether you're new or experienced, there's always something new to discover. We evolve over time, adding new knowledge and letting go of what no longer serves us. In the end, every practitioner builds a practice that is unique to them, shaped by their interests, needs, skills, and experiences.

And here is my point, finally: Understanding the principles of folk magic and spell crafting will allow you to surpass the "following the recipe" phase of your practice and catapult you into the creative stream where one brings elements together intellectually, intuitively, and inspirationally to effect change.

I want to start by talking about the basic qualities I believe are essential to being a folk witch. This point might seem obvious, but I'll say it anyway: You have to believe in magic and in yourself. Magic is real and accessible to anyone who chooses to work with it. So, what is magic? Magic is the neutral energy that connects the seen and unseen worlds, much like electricity. We can't see electricity, but we can feel it and see how it powers a light bulb. Magic works in a similar way—it's all around us, and belief in yourself helps you break through any limitations and tap into that energy.

Learn

It's important to educate yourself and be open to learning. We're living in an incredible time when access to knowledge is easier than ever. There are countless books on witchcraft, folk magic, and related subjects like herbalism and astrology. Folk magic has become so mainstream that you can find resources all over the Internet—through podcasts, videos, and the social media accounts of practicing folk witches. Not all the information out there is correct or accurate, however. The more you learn, the better you'll become at discerning if the information you are ingesting is based in real folk magic or just a performance. Learning also brings discernment to be able to understand what practices resonate with you. It's also valuable to study the history, customs, and folklore of your ancestors. If you live in a place different from where your ancestors came from, take time to learn about the traditions of that area too. A lot of folk magic is tied to the local customs and folklore of specific regions, and understanding them can deepen your practice.

Gain Knowledge of Your Craft

Understanding your craft comes from more than just reading about it. It involves exploring related subjects that can deepen your practice. For folk magic, this includes areas like herbalism, local folklore, the history and geography of the land where the practice is rooted, politics, language, customs, and traditions. These subjects help enrich your understanding of folk magic and its context. We're not born knowing everything, so it's important to actively seek knowledge and, when possible, find a mentor. It's unrealistic to think that reading just one introductory book makes you an expert, but that book can be the starting point for something much larger—opening up new ideas and possibilities. Read widely, listen to experienced practitioners, soak up as much information as you can, and don't be afraid to ask questions. Get hands-on experience and engage fully in your craft. Be open-minded, but also take the time to form your own conclusions. The most important thing is not just acquiring knowledge, but also truly understanding the principles behind it. Once you grasp those, you'll be able to adapt and practice with whatever resources are available to you.

Trust Your Instincts

We all have gut feelings, and they're built into us for a reason—survival. No matter how things look on the outside, if something feels off, trust that feeling. Even if physical evidence suggests that everything is fine, if your gut says otherwise, listen to it. If you feel drawn to do something, follow that energy. Whether it's deciding whom to trust or picking an ingredient for a spell, learn to follow your instincts. They'll never lead you astray.

Meditate

Learn to clear your mind and focus on a single thought. Whether it's the noise from others or your own inner chatter, the goal is to quiet that noise so you can make space for the thoughts and ideas you want to explore. I used to struggle with meditation until I found methods that worked for me. We're all different, and what works for one person may not work for another. For me, journaling helps clear my mind. Journaling is the way I empty the noise in my mind onto paper. I write down everything—no matter how small or big the thoughts are. Sometimes it's just a sentence; other times, it's five pages. Once I get it all on paper, I feel lighter, and my mind becomes quiet. I discard the journaling by burning when possible or shredding. Then, I focus on one idea to meditate on. Sometimes, I sit quietly and ponder a thought, often philosophical or spiritual. Other times, I use something visual, like watching birds in the trees, to help me focus as I reflect on what freedom means to me.

Visualization: A Key Skill in Magic and Ritual

One of the most invaluable skills in spell work and rituals is the ability to visualize. In witchcraft we often hear how crucial it is to form a strong, clear mental image in our mind of what we wish to accomplish or bring forth when performing magic and rituals. Visualization is not just about seeing something in your mind; it is about focusing your intent, directing your energy, and aligning your thoughts with your desired outcome. By clearly envisioning your goal, you set in motion a chain of events within yourself. Your subconscious mind begins to work toward that goal, subtly guiding you to take the necessary steps in the mundane world to bring it to fruition. In this way, visualization acts as a bridge between intention and action, between thought and physical form. Visualization is also the primary way we can receive messages from our spirits.

Overcoming Challenges with Visualization

Not everyone experiences visualization in the same way. Some people experience aphantasia, in which the brain doesn't form or use mental images as part of thinking or imagination. Another way of putting it is the inability to picture in the mind. Aphantasia is not a medical condition, disorder, or disability. Instead, it's a characteristic, much like which hand is your dominant hand. I have partial aphantasia, which means my ability to form mental images is not always or completely absent. It is inconsistent. Sometimes I can picture things in my mind, and other times, especially during times of high stress and exhaustion, I cannot. Sometimes, it is completely random. For those of us with aphantasia (whether partial or complete), traditional visualization techniques may not be consistent or possible at all. Even when I'm not experiencing aphantasia, I rely on my other senses for "visualization" in my practice; it's simply a habit. I use sound, touch, taste, and smell as natural supports to guide my magical work, and this is just how I've always done it. I am not limited by aphantasia because my other senses are always there to support me, regardless of whether I'm actively experiencing it or not. When I'm not experiencing aphantasia, the ability to see in my mind's eye is a bonus, but I still rely on my other senses as my main tools for visualization and connection.

Through trial and experience, I've developed alternative strategies that work for me (and for others I've shared them with), helping me engage with my intentions in a tangible, sensory way. If you struggle with mental imagery, you might find these methods helpful too:

Write it down: Instead of visualizing, describe in vivid detail what you wish to call into being. Write in the present tense—what does it look like, feel like, smell like? The more details, the better.

Create art: If words don't feel right, try expressing your intention through drawing, painting, sculpting, or even digital art. The act of physically crafting something that represents your goal can be just as effective as mental visualization. I have found that this approach is even better.

Make a vision board: A classic technique, a vision board is a collage of images, words, and symbols that represent what you want to bring into your life. You can use magazines, printed images, or even digital tools to create a powerful visual representation of your desires.

Construct a 3D model: Go beyond flat images and create something more interactive. A small-scale model, a physical symbol, or especially a handcrafted item infused with your intent can help you connect with your goal in a tangible way.

Build dioramas: One of my personal favorites, a diorama is a miniature scene that represents my desired outcome. Your scene could be as simple or as elaborate as you like. What matters is that it serves as a focal point for your energy and intent.

Regardless of the method you choose, the most important part is to dedicate uninterrupted time each day to engage with your visualization—whether it's through writing, art, or physical objects. Make it a ritual to connect with your goal and reinforce your intent.

Magic is not about fitting into a one-size-fits-all mold. It's about finding what works for you. Even if you cannot "see" your desired outcome in your mind's eye, you can see the physical representations you created and thus manifest it through other sensory and creative means. What matters is intention, belief, and action.

Emotions

Emotions are key in working magic. It's important to be aware of and, as much as possible, in control of our emotions, especially for folk magicians. In my culture, there's a belief that when glass shatters without reason, "a witch did it"—suggesting it's an intentional energetic attack. But in my experience, this phenomenon was different. Someone I knew with a very volatile temperament—someone who could go from calm to furious in an instant—left a trail of destruction when they lost their temper. Glasses drying in the dish rack would shatter, light bulbs would break, picture frames would fall. Rage, in this case, was a powerful and uncontrollable force. But imagine the potential if that person could harness that energy and direct it with focus and precision.

Knowing yourself is crucial because understanding your strongest, most primal emotion unlocks your magical power. Intention is the spark, and emotion is the accelerant. What is your strongest emotion? Is it fear, shame, panic, rage, joy, or ecstasy? Mastering the ability to harness powerful emotions—especially those commonly viewed as destructive—requires maturity, self-awareness, and practice. Be patient with yourself; this is a lifelong process. Grounding exercises or rituals are helpful during times of intense emotions. You can ground by physically touching the earth, moving your body, or taking care of yourself, by nourishing your body or taking a bath. Also, think back to when you were a child. Where would you hide when you were afraid? What comforted you?

Stewardship

Stewardship of our environment, both seen and unseen, is about the careful and responsible management of everything entrusted to our care. This applies to ourselves, the people and animals we care for, the land we live on, the spirits we connect with, and our environment as a whole. A good example of stewardship is taking care of our home—not just the physical structure we live in, but also the people, pets, and spirits that share that space, as well as the surrounding land and nature. The most important part of stewardship, however, is managing our own personal resources—our health and fitness, both physical and emotional, psychological, and spiritual—and the health and fitness of all beings in our care. Stewardship also involves the responsible management of resources. Folk magic, rooted in the practices of ordinary people with little to no resources, emphasizes using what you have, taking only what you need, being respectful, and avoiding wastefulness.

Help without Doing

Being willing to help but not do the work for others is an important balance. Helping can mean listening while someone processes their emotions, offering advice when asked, or simply holding space for someone going through a tough time. It's natural for friends and family to turn to us, wanting us to fix things for them. In those situations, I help by guiding them to help themselves. People tend to value things more when they've put in the effort themselves, and this applies to both magic and life. I'm always ready to help remove the evil eye or offer spiritual support, but the work of healing or change is ultimately theirs to do. There have been rare instances when I've felt it was appropriate to cast a spell on someone's behalf, but these are few and far between. As I mentioned earlier, magic comes at a price. That price could be a loss in exchange for a gain, or it might be my old nemesis—the unintended consequence. Every decision we make and every action we take have consequences, and some of these consequences are unintended. Folk magic is no exception; it's not immune to those unintended outcomes.

Let me give you a relatable example. Let's say you're behind on paying your bills, and your family depends on you. You cast a spell to find work and apply for a job. You're interviewed, but you're not sure how you did. You stay hopeful and keep feeding your spell. Ten days later, you get a call—praise the spirits, you got the job! Your new employer tells you they were going to offer it to someone else, but that candidate fell down a flight of stairs and broke their back. Now, as long as you're ready to work, the job is yours.

Did your spell work? Yes. Did you intend harm? No. But could your spell have had something to do with the accident? Possibly. That person was the first choice, and now, due to their misfortune, the job is yours. This might be an unintended consequence of your spell.

Without the spell, the situation could have just been random chance, where the other candidate's bad luck worked in your favor. But you know you cast the spell. Some folk witches approach magic with the understanding that there may be unintended consequences, and they hope those consequences are harmless. Magic always has a price, whether we realize it or not.

Folk witches understand the costs associated with magic. We don't shy away from baneful magic; instead, we use whatever resources we have to remove obstacles between us and our goals, whether that's benign magic, baneful magic, or anything in between. Each witch has their own morals and ethics. What's important is knowing where we stand, being true to ourselves, and being accountable for our actions.

To be an effective and well-rounded witch, we need to understand all sides of magic. We must know how harm is inflicted in order to be good healers. We need to understand curses—the components, actions, and the spirits involved. Without this knowledge, we can never effectively diagnose or remove a curse. It's dangerous and foolish to think otherwise.

This is why I am always available to advise and consult on what actions may be taken, but I will not do the magical work on behalf of another person (except in very rare and specific circumstances). This is my personal choice. It is not reflective of every other folk magician. Nor am I passing judgment on anyone who does sell spell-casting services.

The beauty of practicing folk magic is we are all free to practice as we see fit. We are also free to change our minds at any time. When it comes to our personal practice, we make the rules, and we are free to change those rules at any given moment.

Contagion, a principle in sympathetic magic, involves two types: imitative and contagious magic. Imitative magic is based on the idea that "like attracts like." Essentially, the effect mirrors the cause. For example, if a magician wants to harm an enemy, they might injure an image or representation of that enemy, believing the injury will affect the person. It can also be seen as creating a small-scale version of what you intend to manifest on a larger scale. Contagious magic is rooted in the belief that once something was part of a person or object, it remains connected to that original thing, even at a distance. Any action performed on the part (such as hair or nails) will affect the person it came from. This concept is widely believed across various cultures. A common example is the superstition that possessing someone's hair or nails allows one to influence that person from afar.

I love sympathetic magic because it's simple, quick, and can be done anywhere with minimal supplies. It's elegant in its simplicity. For example, one way of using the element of water to "cool them down" is to place a name or item belonging to someone who is targeting us into a container of water and freeze it. As the water freezes around the object, the person's anger or aggression is subdued. Even nonpractitioners can understand this, as the spell relies on the basic concept of changing a state of being, not necessarily belief in the spirit of water. This principle works anywhere and anytime, as long as you understand the energetic properties of your desired outcome. For instance, placing a photo or names of a quarreling couple into a jar of honey to "sweeten" their relationship is another example. This technique can be applied to any relationship—friends, business partners, family, and more.

In contagious magic, objects that have made physical contact with one another can transfer energy or essence, creating a permanent link. Once in contact, they remain connected. For example, the sweet properties of honey transferred to a quarreling couple can help them "sweeten" toward each other. This is why my Neapolitan relatives were protective of their fingernail trimmings and hair clippings, as these items carry the essence of the person they were once attached to. Another example is how food, prepared with love, carries the energy of the person who made it, making it taste better.

Another type of sympathetic magic, and arguably the type most commonly practiced by most people in every culture, is apotropaic magic, whether or not other kinds of magic are practiced. Apotropaic, also known as protective magic, is a form of magic designed to ward off harm or negative influences, such as deflecting misfortune or preventing the effects of the evil eye. Apotropaic practices often include good luck charms and amulets most commonly in the form of charm bracelets, necklaces, and keychains and such. Examples of apotropaic charms are the rabbit's foot, holed stone also known as hag stone, bindrune (a symbol made up of two or more Nordic runes), the nazar (eye-shaped amulet made of blue glass), Norwegian and Swedish trollkors (Troll Cross), and symbolic gestures like crossing fingers or knocking on wood. Various objects and charms have been used for protection throughout history, and they continue to be used today.

Speak Intentionally

Words matter deeply to me. As a writer, I understand their power, but my connection to words goes beyond my profession. Growing up, I was raised by people who were very careful with their words because they believed that words were spells. They feared speaking the wrong words, thinking they could inadvertently cast negative magic. I have seen firsthand how words can hold power, which is why I am precise with mine. The word *intention* has been overused in mainstream culture to the point that its true meaning has been diluted. It's often used as a stand-in for *spell*, *magic*, or *witchcraft*, losing much of its weight. But to me, intention is everything. It is the driving force behind every action. Intention is both the beginning and the end of magic. It's the will we put forth, the will we call into the world.

This will resides in the area of our body known as the solar plexus, located between the chest and the pelvis. It's the center of our physical being, and for those familiar with the chakra system, it corresponds to the third chakra. You may wonder why I'm focusing on this part of the body. Here's why: True intention doesn't come from the mind. The mind may form the idea, but the power to manifest it is born in the solar plexus. Intention starts as a seed in the mind, and that idea is nurtured and transformed into action in the solar plexus. It is the heart's wish that fuels the power to bring the idea into being. When you truly want something, you can feel it deep in your body.

Sympathetic Magic and Desire

Sympathetic magic operates on the principle of "like attracts like," where our desires and gratitude serve as powerful catalysts. The best time to apply sympathetic magic is when we're directly experiencing what we want or a close version of it. Being able to touch, see, or feel that thing we desire in the moment allows us to anchor that desire in the present, fueling it with excitement and joy. If we see someone else in a situation we desire, instead of feeling envious, we should cultivate true happiness for their good fortune. This sincerity helps bring that fortune into our own lives. I view this process as a metaphorical garment. When I see someone else in a favorable situation, I imagine that situation fitting me perfectly. I don that metaphorical garment, and with all my senses, I fully experience how right it feels. I then release the desire, trusting that it will manifest when the time is right.

This process, which bridges the tangible and intangible, is about transforming a wish into intention through the solar plexus, where the desire becomes a physical sensation. It's about trusting that what belongs to us is already on its way. The key to manifestation is a deep longing coupled with faith—faith that something or someone is listening and willing to help us. When we long for something, we're connecting with what's meant for us, whether it's relationships, status, or success. That deep longing, felt in every fiber of our being, is the energy we need to send our request into the universe. Whether it's called a spell or a prayer, the act is the same: It's a sincere, heartfelt wish that aligns us with what we desire. Through synchronicities and signs, the universe begins to move us closer to our goals.

Openness

Always be learning, growing, and exploring. Keep your heart and mind open. I've long stopped labeling myself or my practice because it's limiting. Magic is multifaceted, and no label can capture every aspect of it. While labels can help connect us with like-minded people, they can also be restrictive or just a trend. Not everyone who uses the same label practices the same way or feels the same connection. We are all unique, so labels often don't do us justice.

Recently, I've noticed people labeling themselves based on what's trending on social media, often without fully understanding what that label means or what it entails. How can you label yourself when you haven't yet explored what truly resonates with you? For example, if someone claims to be a green witch but has no passion for plants, what happens when they realize the label of green witch doesn't align with who they are?

Stay open, my friends. Stay open to new experiences, ideas, and paradigms. Be willing to change your mind when presented with new evidence. Let your practice evolve as you grow. Stay open to releasing what no longer serves you and welcoming the new. When we stay open, we become malleable and elastic, allowing the energy and experiences to flow freely, as we dance through the universe.

Survival Skills

Basic survival skills are essential tools in your personal arsenal. Take up hobbies that once were crucial skills our ancestors had to know. Sewing, crocheting, knitting, woodworking, gardening, cooking, baking, food preservation, winemaking, beer brewing, first aid, basic veterinary care, homemaking, house maintenance, and the ability to repair things—these are just a few examples. These hobbies are more than just activities; they are life skills that promote independence.

Embracing a do-it-yourself (DIY) lifestyle is empowering. The more skills we acquire, the more self-sufficient and free we become. There's a unique satisfaction in learning to create or fix something yourself. The things we make carry our energy and magic, connecting us to our work in a way that's meaningful. The desire to take control of our environment through these skills mirrors the drive to take control of our lives in the magical sense. While we can't control everything, we can work to maintain stability.

We are fortunate to have a vast amount of information at our fingertips. With a simple Internet search, we can find detailed instructions and tutorials on almost anything—especially from YouTube channels dedicated to these old-fashioned but invaluable skills.

Learning the skills our ancestors relied on for survival not only brings us closer to them but also empowers us. Countless times, I've set out to learn a new skill, whether it's cooking a dish I've never made before or tackling a home repair, and felt the presence of my ancestors guiding me. As I work, I begin to feel like I instinctively know what I'm doing. And when I'm done, I look at my creation or repair in awe, realizing I accomplished it all by myself without prior knowledge or experience.

Know Your Limitations and Use That Awareness to Focus on Your Strengths

Focus on what you're passionate about and master it. For example, I'm not a green witch, but I'm deeply knowledgeable about the plants I work with in my magic. I understand their scientific, medicinal, and magical properties, and I have long-standing relationships with their spirits. I stick to the plants I know, growing or foraging as much as I can. However, that doesn't mean I'm an expert in every plant.

Similarly, I have a working knowledge of astrology, particularly lunar and planetary correspondences, but I'm not an astrologer. Astrology is part of my practice, although I don't know how to read my own chart. I focus on the parts of astrology that serve me and keep notes in my grimoire for things I need to reference.

When I first started my magical journey, I was a voracious learner, eager to know everything. But realistically, I can't know everything or be an expert in everything. There simply aren't enough hours in the day to incorporate every subject into my practice. I've learned to accept that I won't be the best at everything, but I can always strive to give my best to everything I do.

Understanding our limitations allows us to specialize and focus on our strengths. Once we do that, we can expand our knowledge in areas that truly ignite our passion. Awareness of our limitations gives us limitless potential in the areas where we can excel.

Understand Yourself

Are you a group person or solitary? Both have their pros and cons. Personally, I'm firmly solitary and introverted, but even as a solitary folk practitioner, I believe community is important. However, the type of community you connect with will look different depending on whether you're more group-oriented or solitary. A group person would likely be drawn to covens and group rituals, focusing on a coven-style witchcraft practice rather than folk witchery. In contrast, a solitary practitioner is more likely to be drawn to folk practices, which are inherently solitary, but also benefit from close ties with other solitary practitioners. Some people find a balance, practicing both. For example, my friend was part of a Wiccan coven but also practiced folk magic outside of it. As a solitary practitioner, I deeply cherish the intimate relationships I have with other solitary kindreds. The exchange of ideas and experiences between us is invaluable, and I love the cross-pollination of our practices that comes from these connections. If you're unsure which type of practice suits you best, there's only one way to find out: Try different things until you feel at home and discover what feels most natural to you.

Be in Your Body

Understand your physical environment, and that includes your body. Being truly in tune with your body means recognizing what it feels like when you're in a state of well-being, both physically and energetically. When you know what your baseline of wellness feels like, you can easily notice when something shifts. Our bodies serve as a defense against both the physical and spiritual/psychic realms. Unusual sensations can signal that we are picking up psychic information, interference, or even an attack. Learn to listen to your body. Its feedback can help you identify symptoms, such as those related to the evil eye or spiritual imbalances. Your body acts as a messenger, alerting you when the magical remedies you've implemented either are working or need to be repeated. It can also act as radar, letting you know when spirits are nearby, warning you if they are trustworthy or if they carry a potential threat.

A good place to begin is cultivating awareness of how your body feels in its normal state and learning to interpret the messages it sends. We are embodied spirits, and our body is the vessel through which we experience and engage with the world. Sensations in our bodies can alert us to physical illness through symptoms or danger through experiences like goosebumps or the hairs standing up on the back of our necks. That gut feeling of unease literally comes from a physical sensation in your stomach when something feels wrong. By truly knowing your body, you strengthen your ability to develop intuition and trust your instincts. This self-awareness is vital for decision-making and invaluable when interacting with people or spirits. When you're in tune with your body, you'll be able to detect even the most subtle changes. For example, I can instantly feel when a spirit is near; it's like a warm blanket being draped over my shoulders or a gentle hand resting on my head. This physical awareness is an essential tool in connecting with the energies and spirits around us.

Be True to Yourself

The phrase "be true to yourself" has become so overused that it often sounds like a cliché, so obvious that it's easy to gloss over or dismiss. But the truth is, it's overused because it holds a deep, timeless wisdom. I've come to truly appreciate how profound the meaning behind this message really is. It's not just a feel-good statement; it's essential to our survival and well-being. Yet, as much as I strive to be true to myself, I'll admit that it's incredibly challenging to maintain this consistency all the time. Being true to yourself means rejecting anything that doesn't align with your inner experience—your motives, beliefs, values, ethics, morals, and personal disposition. But, let's be real: It's hard work. It's a constant effort . . . and a full-time job on top of just surviving. The truth is, I've had varying levels of success with being self-aware and staying true to myself, in both the short and long term. It's a continual process, and it's always a work in progress. The reason it's so difficult is that both the world around us and we ourselves are always changing.

In times of change, insight often feels fleeting and hard to grasp. What I've learned, however, is that there's a happy medium: Be true to yourself as best you can, right in this present moment. Take one moment at a time. The truth is, your practice, your journey, is between you and yourself, and you and your spirits. Nothing else matters more than that. This journey is about staying grounded in who you are, adjusting as needed, and not beating yourself up for not having it all figured out.

Maintain Accountability

Accountability is a cornerstone of both personal growth and magical practice. We all make mistakes. It's part of being human, and we all sometimes make the wrong decisions. But what sets us apart is how we respond. Being accountable for our actions, especially when they lead to unintended consequences, is a vital part of learning and evolving. In the realm of folk magic, this means owning both the successes and the failures of our practices, and not shying away from the responsibility of what we've set into motion. When we are accountable for our actions, we are acknowledging our role in the outcomes, whether positive or negative. This act of owning our decisions opens us up to receiving help, guidance, and wisdom from those around us—whether that be from fellow practitioners, ancestors, spirits, or simply the lessons embedded in our experiences. Accountability creates a space where we can learn, grow, and correct our course when things don't go as planned. Correcting course is especially important when dealing with unintended consequences in our magical workings. Magic is a force that often moves in ways we can't always predict, and sometimes, we find ourselves facing results we didn't anticipate. But if we approach those results with a mindset of accountability—acknowledging our part, reflecting on what happened, and being willing to make adjustments—we can transform those missteps into valuable lessons. We can shift our focus from blame to understanding, from frustration to solution, and in doing so, we become more effective and responsible practitioners.

In the end, accountability is not just about recognizing when we've gone astray; it's about embracing the process of course correction, learning from our mistakes, and becoming more attuned to the ebb and flow of our magical work. This effort, in turn, helps us grow as people and as practitioners of folk magic.

Curse to Heal

To be truly effective at countering curses, a folk witch must first understand how they work—in both mechanics and intent. Just as a healer must know the nature of a disease to cure it, a practitioner of folk magic must recognize the structure of a curse to dismantle it. This means understanding how energy, intent, and symbolic action interact to bind, afflict, or manipulate fate. Knowing how to curse teaches the practitioner not only how harm is inflicted but also how it can be unraveled—whether through reversal, purification, or redirection. Without this knowledge, breaking a hex is like attempting to disarm a trap blindfolded. The folk witch's role is not just to heal but also to restore balance, and sometimes that requires wielding the same forces they seek to neutralize.

> *Have more than you show,*
> *Speak less than you know.*
>
> —William Shakespeare

The wise old ones always said that the best shield against envy and the evil eye is to maintain a low profile. They cautioned against broadcasting our accomplishments, our good fortune, and always encouraged projecting humility and discretion. "You never know who is watching you with jealousy and envy in their hearts, wishing you harm," they warned. In those days, privacy was a matter of course; nowadays, in a world where nearly everyone is broadcasting their private lives, it feels as though the rules have changed. With witchcraft becoming more mainstream, many practitioners now share their practices on social media. It's so easy and so tempting to get swept up in the "witchy purple haze" and join the online show-and-tell. I don't take issue with that; I actually think it can be quite fun, as long as it's done safely. Sharing your favorite media, divination tools, witchy aesthetic, crafts, and hobbies is, in my view, perfectly safe. However, I do stand firm on two things that I will never share: my actual magical workings—real spells and rituals in progress—and the identities of the spirits in my spirit court.

I am more than happy to demonstrate how to perform a magical working for educational purposes, and I love discussing spirits and their roles in our practices. But there's a fine line between sharing what you are passionate about and sharing the intimate details of your personal magical practice and relationships with spirits. For me, that line is nonnegotiable. The wise ones taught me well: "You never know who is watching and listening," especially on the Internet. You don't know who your rivals are or how sharing intimate information might come back to negatively affect you or those you care about. Keeping certain aspects of your practice and spirit relationships private is a form of protection. It's a way to safeguard yourself, your energy, and your work. As people say, "Loose lips sink ships." It's a lesson that remains as relevant today as it was back then. When we choose to keep some things to ourselves, we are creating a boundary that allows us to stay safe, grounded, and protected in our magical lives.

Mind Your Own Business

Avoid insinuating yourself into another's situation under the guise of being helpful. The truth is, there's no such thing as a completely selfless act, no matter how much we might convince ourselves otherwise. We may want to help, but often our desire to assist comes with a certain degree of ego. I'm approachable, and I'm always open to offering help and advice when someone asks for it, but I will never assume that I know what's best for someone else or impose my "help" upon them. When you offer unsolicited help, especially when it's unwelcome or unnecessary, it's not only an invasion of their privacy, it's also an overstep of their boundaries. It's a subtle way of saying, "I know what's best for you," without considering whether that's true or whether they even want or need help. More often than not, this kind of behavior feeds our own ego rather than serving the other person. It's a delicate balance to maintain: We must honor others' autonomy and their ability to handle their own problems in their own way. Think of it this way: If you wedge yourself between someone and their problems, those problems become yours. You take on more than what's healthy for you, and you also rob the other person of the agency to navigate their own challenges. That's why I refrain from offering insight or advice on a situation unless it's specifically requested of me. Everyone has their own path, and we should respect their journey. When someone reaches out for guidance, that's when it's appropriate to step in. Until then, it's best to honor their space and trust that they have the strength to handle things in their own time and in their own way.

Not Just a Practice

Folk magic is not just something you practice—it's a way of living. While reading books and observing other people's practices are valuable ways to learn, remember that folk magic requires more than theory. It's a hands-on practice, one that demands you roll up your sleeves and get your hands dirty, both literally and figuratively. It's through doing the work—getting involved in the rituals, the spells, the everyday acts of magic—that we truly learn and grow.

Don't be afraid of failure. Too often, fear of failure paralyzes us, causing us to avoid trying altogether. But failure is one of the most powerful teachers. It shows us what doesn't work and teaches us how to refine our craft. It's in the doing that we hone our skills. The more we practice, the sharper our intuition becomes. The more we engage with our work, the more confident we grow in our abilities.

Seeking feedback from others, sharing experiences, and learning from fellow practitioners—especially the cross-pollination of different cultural practices, superstitions, and beliefs—enrich us all. When we share what we know, we all grow. We all benefit. Folk magic thrives in community, even when that community is made up of solitary practitioners who share a love for learning, exchanging ideas, and experimenting. So, roll up your sleeves and get into it. Put into practice what you have learned and don't let the fear of making mistakes stop you from branching out. When we're new to something, we often believe that even the smallest mistake will lead to catastrophe. But as we continue practicing, we become comfortable and set in our ways. We might avoid trying new things because we've become complacent, but that's when our practices risk stagnation. Welcome change into your life and practice. It keeps everything fresh, dynamic, and growing. We're constantly evolving, and it's only natural that our magical practices must evolve alongside us. Most of the time, change brings growth and rejuvenation, but sometimes, the new thing doesn't work out the way we expect, or it leads to a completely opposite result from what we wanted. That's life. And it's perfectly fine.

I've made more mistakes than I can count, but every single one of them taught me something invaluable. Mistakes help us correct course, teaching us what to adjust when things don't turn out the way we planned. In some cases, mistakes lead to successful innovation—discovering something entirely new, something that we wouldn't have found if we hadn't dared to make the mistake in the first place.

A folk witch is never idle. We don't wait for magic to happen; we make it happen. Whether it's preparing food, caring for our environment, or working at a job—no matter what the occupation—there's always magic in what we do. A folk witch cannot stop witching, because witchcraft isn't a practice that lives in isolation. It's woven into everything we do. It's in the way we approach life, in how we shape our world, in every action we take. For a folk witch, magic is not a task—it's a natural state of being.

The Value of Divination Skills in Folk Magic

Divination is deeply woven into the fabric of folk magic. The word itself comes from the Latin *divinare*, meaning "to predict." According to the *Merriam-Webster* dictionary, divination is "the art or practice that seeks to foresee or foretell future events or discover hidden knowledge, usually by the interpretation of omens or by the aid of supernatural powers" (*www.merriam-webster.com*). However, what this definition doesn't fully capture is that divination also involves using divinatory tools—like tarot cards, runes, pendulums, or tea leaves—to uncover hidden truths or glimpse future events.

Divination, or fortune-telling, was, for me, the entry point into my magical practice. It's often how many of us are first drawn to this way of life. The tools of divination, whether they are physical like cards or runes or something more abstract like intuition, act as gateways to the spirit world. They provide a way to interpret symbols, omens, or messages from beyond the veil. These tools can act as intermediaries, guiding us to hidden knowledge or offering glimpses of what's yet to come.

I've met countless people who practice some form of divination—be it through cards, pendulums, tea leaves, or other methods—who will claim they don't practice folk magic. This sentiment is common, and while they may not be casting spells or performing rituals in the traditional sense, what they are doing when they engage with divination is, in essence, a form of magical practice. Even though they might not label it as such, the act of using divinatory tools to access hidden knowledge or predict the future is a form of spirit work. They are tapping into the unseen, seeking answers that are not readily available through the physical senses.

When you read cards or tea leaves, or look to the stars, or cast bones, you're engaging with the spirit world—whether you realize it or not. The tools serve as a means to interpret symbols, which are believed to be arranged by spirits to reveal information that is hidden or not yet made known. These symbols, often seen as omens or messages, carry layers of meaning and insight, and through interpretation, the diviner is able to decode the messages. Whether it's insight into a personal situation or a glimpse into a possible future, divination bridges the gap between the physical and spiritual realms. So, even if one does not consciously identify as practicing folk magic, anyone who seeks answers or insights through divination is, in effect, participating in a form of magical work. I can't imagine how a folk witch would even communicate with their spirits without being skilled in divination. It's a way of communicating with the unseen forces around us, asking questions, and receiving guidance through the language of symbols, omens, and intuition.

Spirits in Folk Magic

Spirits are at the heart of folk magic. While folk magic itself is not a religion, it is deeply rooted in a relationship with the spirit world. It's more about living in communion with the unseen, the energies, forces, and entities beyond our immediate physical reality, than adhering to a specific set of religious doctrines. You do not need to believe in any gods or follow any particular religion to practice folk magic. However, many practitioners incorporate religious texts, symbols, or iconography into their practices—things that hold personal meaning and connect them to the spirit world. This connection to the spiritual realm is what makes folk magic alive and dynamic.

Folk magic is an art—a practice that is highly adaptable to the cultural and religious background of the practitioner. It's shaped by what resonates with you and the traditions you choose to follow. Whether you're steeped in the folklore of your ancestors, drawing on the practices of different cultures (incorporating your ancestral culture and the culture of where you were born), or creating something entirely unique, folk magic is about working with the energies around you, including the spirits that inhabit these realms. It is my firm belief—and my experience—that you can practice folk magic without adhering to a formal religion, but you cannot practice it without acknowledging and engaging with the spirit world. Spirits are the unseen partners in our magical work. Whether or not we actively acknowledge them or choose to cultivate relationships with them, they are the ones responding when we engage in magic or ritual. Once you accept that the spirit world is actively involved in your practice, you open the door to deeper communication. Spirits are not passive; they respond to your intent, your work, and your energy. They are present, and once you begin to recognize their presence, you can start to communicate with them—whether through divination, ritual, or even simply through the subtle feelings, sensations, and signs they offer. Building relationships with these spirits can be mutually beneficial, enriching both your spiritual practice and your everyday life.

Folk magic thrives on the exchange between the practitioner and the spirits. It's a two-way relationship—one that requires respect, awareness, and communication. The more you engage with the spirit world, the more you realize how much the spirits enrich and guide your practice. They can offer wisdom, protection, and assistance, and as you develop these connections, you'll find that your magical work becomes more focused, more potent, and more aligned with your needs and desires. The spirit world is not just a part of folk magic. It is the very force that powers it.

When I first started down the path of witchcraft, I had a very simple and somewhat naive understanding of magic. In my youth, I fully bought into the idea of "I am the magic." I believed that witchcraft was akin to cooking, where you just follow a recipe and, as long as you follow the steps correctly, you'll get the desired result. This mindset worked for me early on, but not necessarily in the way I thought. My very first experience with casting a spell came through my Cuban immigrant neighbor, who shared a spell with me. (I have included this spell in the grimoire section at the back of this book.) I was eager to try it, and so I followed the instructions carefully. I gathered all the required items, read the incantation aloud just as I was told, and awaited the results. To my utter surprise, I was absolutely stunned when the spell worked almost instantly. My problem was resolved, and I was ecstatic. Everything unfolded just as I had hoped.

What I didn't realize at the time was that this spell wasn't just a series of words and objects. Embedded in the incantation was an evocation to a spirit—one from my neighbor's cultural and magical tradition that I wasn't familiar with. The spell was not just a mechanical process; it was a connection to something deeper, something beyond my immediate understanding. To explain it more simply, imagine a phone number. My neighbor had referred me to someone they knew and trusted—a spirit who dealt with the issue that was troubling me. By giving me the spell, they were essentially providing me with the phone number to reach this spirit. I "dialed the number" correctly by following the spell, and the spirit answered the call, granting me the help I needed.

Looking back, I see that this experience was a significant moment in my magical journey. It taught me an important lesson: Witchcraft is not just about following a set of instructions. It's about invoking, connecting with, and working with forces beyond the material world. At that time, I had no idea what I was doing beyond following the spell, but I received the benefit because the spirit responded. Now, with more experience, I understand that magic is not just about following a formula. It's about the relationships you build with the spiritual and unseen forces, and how you learn to call on them, work with them, and respect their power. That first spell, though it was simple, opened my eyes to the deeper, more profound elements of witchcraft that would continue to shape my path.

Interacting with spirits is a lot like interacting with the living. Suppose you need help with something, like accomplishing a project or completing a task. Naturally, you would reach out to someone you believe is capable of assisting you. After you ask, it's up to that person to decide if they can and will help you. Let's say they agree to assist. In return, you express your gratitude by doing something kind for them, like buying them a coffee or offering your help should they ever need it. This mutual exchange makes it more likely that they will offer their help again when needed. Now, let's apply this same concept to spirits. Just as with a living person, spirits have their own will, personality, and preferences. When you reach out to a spirit for help, you are making a request, but the spirit ultimately decides whether or not they wish to assist you. This is why respect, proper offerings, and gratitude are so important in spirit work. It's not a matter of demanding help, but rather inviting it, recognizing that their assistance is a gift.

For this example, let's say you're seeking help in finding gainful employment. You decide to approach Freyr, the Norse god of prosperity, abundance, and good harvests, who is often associated with bringing favorable results in matters of wealth and career. Freyr, like all spirits, can be called on to help you achieve your goals, but he will assist based on the respect and energy you put into your request.

Here's a basic formula for reaching out to Freyr, though this framework can be adapted for any spirit and any request.

Step-by-Step Guide

1. Prepare Offerings

Offerings are an important part of the ritual. They are your way of showing respect to the spirit you are asking for help from. In the case of Freyr, offerings such as bread, alcohol made from grains, and honey are traditional and symbolic of abundance. You can offer one or several of these items based on what feels right, but the key is that the offering should be the best you have or can afford in the moment.

2. Choose a Quiet, Uninterrupted Time and Place

Select a space where you won't be disturbed and can fully focus on your connection with the spirit. This could be at an altar, a special spot in your home, or any place that feels sacred to you.

3. Introduce Yourself to the Spirit

When you're working with a spirit for the first time, it's important to introduce yourself and clearly state your intention. For example:

> "My name is [Your Name], and I ask Freyr, Norse god of prosperity and abundance, to bless me with gainful employment."

4. Make the Offering

Place your offering (in this case, the loaf of bread) on your table or altar. As you do, say something like:

> "Thank you, Freyr, for all your gifts. I offer this as a token of my gratitude."

Then leave the offering undisturbed, trusting that the spirit has received your request.

5. Follow Through in the Physical World

While you're engaging with the spirit world, don't forget the practical steps required to manifest your goal. For a job search, this means actively applying for jobs, preparing for interviews, and doing everything you can in the physical world to achieve your goal.

6. Give Thanks after Receiving Help

Once you receive the help you've asked for (in this case, a new job), it's important to take a moment to thank the spirit and make another offering as a gesture of appreciation. You might choose to offer something more or repeat your initial offering, showing that you recognize the exchange and are grateful for their support.

The Role of Relationships with Spirits

Building relationships with spirits is not just about asking for favors. It's about creating a bond over time through trust, respect, and gratitude. Over time, you begin to understand how these exchanges work and what the spirit values. This mutual exchange of energy is the heart of magical practice; it's not just about getting what you want but also about offering something meaningful in return. This process has taught me something incredibly valuable: I am not the center of the universe. I am not entitled to a spirit's assistance, nor should I take their help for granted. Spirit work is an exchange—one that requires both sides to give and take. The energy of magic comes at a cost, and that cost might not always be what you expect.

Let's say Freyr blesses you with the dream job you've been hoping for, but there's a catch. The job requires you to relocate to a city hundreds of miles away, and you'll be far from your friends, family, and familiar surroundings. This is the cost of the exchange—an unforeseen consequence that might push you out of your comfort zone.

But here's the key lesson: All magic has a cost. Whether it's an unexpected sacrifice, a change in circumstances, or a challenge that forces you to grow, there is always a trade-off. The benefit of receiving spirit assistance is balanced by the responsibility of accepting whatever consequences come with it. By building respectful, reciprocal relationships with spirits, you gain wisdom not just in magic, but also in navigating the complexities of life itself.

Our spirits protect and support us. They warn us when something is not right and reveal what is hidden so that we can move forward with our eyes open, allowing us to make more informed decisions about the exchange of energy—the cost—required to achieve our desired outcome. Experience and maturity have taught me that sometimes, no matter how much I want something, the cost may be too high to justify the result.

One of the greatest gifts of developing a solid relationship with your spirits is the reassurance that you are not alone. You will begin to notice evidence of their presence in your life—in small moments, in unexpected solutions to problems you didn't even know existed until they stepped in and resolved them. These moments of quiet intervention deepen the bond between you and your spirits, reinforcing that their guidance is always present, even if you're not always consciously aware of it.

To understand the basic principles of spirit interactions, it helps to recognize that you, too, are a spirit—one currently inhabiting a physical body. Whether you are a beginner or a seasoned practitioner, you may feel like you rarely, if ever, interact with spirits, or that they aren't part of your practice. In truth, this is often a matter of perception rather than a lack of their presence. There have been times when my own life has been so chaotic—especially during periods of stress or worry—that I felt as though my spirits had gone silent or left me altogether. (I will discuss this more in chapter 5.) I don't believe there are strict rules when it comes to interacting with spirits, but there is etiquette. You can begin by forming relationships with the spirits of the formerly living—your ancestors. Ancestors may be connected to you by blood, but they can also be linked through shared profession, location, cultural ties, or personal affinity. Because they were once human, they are often more attuned to our struggles, having experienced the human condition themselves. This familiarity makes it easier for us to approach them, modeling our interactions after the relationships we have with the living.

Since spirits do not have physical form, learning to recognize their presence requires developing an awareness of different energetic signatures. This awareness comes with time and experience. There is no shortcut, but rest assured that even the process of learning is a form of doing. Your spirits are already here, already listening, and as you deepen your connection, you will learn to hear them more clearly.

Chapter 3

Diasporic Folk Magic
History, Spells, and Tools

If we are to preserve culture we must continue to create it.

—Johan Huizinga

Diasporic folk magic refers to the magical traditions, practices, and beliefs that were carried and adapted by immigrants (and their descendants) as they settled in various parts of the world, particularly in regions outside of their native land. These practices often include elements of folk magic, superstitions, rituals, and spiritual beliefs but are shaped and influenced by the new cultures and environments they encountered. The term *diasporic* highlights the experience of people living away from their homeland and the way their magical traditions evolved or merged with other cultural practices in their new homes.

I've met many people from diverse cultures and religions, and we always find common ground when we share our ancestors' immigration stories, traditional foods, proverbs, folklore, customs, and superstitions. While our folktales and symbols may differ, they often share similar themes and characteristics. Ultimately, what unites us is our shared experiences. We all have the same needs and desires, face similar fears and challenges, and confront the same misfortunes in life. To illustrate this, I will share my ancestors' experience.

My practice is deeply rooted in the magical traditions of central and southern Italian immigrants who settled in eastern Canada and the northeastern United States after World War II. The reason is that my family and neighbors came from these regions, bringing their customs, beliefs, and practices with them. When they left their villages, they carried a snapshot of their culture as it existed in that moment—preserved in memory and tradition, even as Italy itself continued to evolve. I cannot begin to imagine what the experience must have been like for them, though I grew up listening to their stories. The stories they chose to tell, that is—the ones suitable for children, appropriate for mixed company. Tales of hardship softened with a heavy dose of "but we were happy."

They left behind everything they had ever known for the complete and utterly terrifying unknown. I often wonder—actually, I still wonder—just how hopeless their post-war situation must have been for them to believe that an uncertain future in a foreign land was still a better option than staying in their homeland. These experiences are not unique to Italian immigrants. They mirror the struggles of countless people across different countries and eras—people forced to leave behind everything familiar in search of something, *anything*, better. Migration, driven by survival, is as old as humanity itself.

Even in today's hyper-connected world, hardship has not been erased. The circumstances may change, but the fundamental choice remains: to step into the unknown, risking everything for the hope of a better life. The people who made that choice were tough, hardworking, and resilient—not because they wanted to be, but because they had no other option. Survival demanded grit, integrity, and an unshakable will. Wherever they settled, they carried their history with them—their language, folklore, customs, religion, superstitions, and fears. They adapted to their new surroundings, but they did not leave behind the beliefs that had shaped their ancestors for generations.

What we now call folk magic was, for them, simply "life." It was their worldview, inseparable from their daily existence. It was in the prayers they whispered, the charms they carried, the rituals they performed to ward off misfortune. It was in the way they honored their dead, sought protection, and called upon unseen forces for guidance. Whether they recognized it as magic or not, their traditions—woven from faith, folklore, and necessity—became the foundation of their lives in a new land.

What we call folk magic and folk witchery today was what these immigrants turned to when all else failed—when there was no other choice.

They turned to it when the doctor couldn't cure them—or when there was no doctor to call.

When the law couldn't (or wouldn't) protect them.

When praying to the God of their church brought no relief.

When they felt their government had abandoned them.

Why? Because it worked.

Even when it didn't work in the way they had hoped, it still did something. It gave them a sense of control, a way to act in a world that often left them powerless. Praying was sometimes not enough. If pressed, they might even admit that prayer alone made them feel subservient, as if they were merely waiting for divine intervention. But charms, incantations, and rituals? Those gave them agency. They weren't just pleading for help; they were taking action, influencing their fate, shaping the outcome as best they could. A protection amulet above the front door was protection—an active barrier against evil. A talisman worn against the skin was safety—a shield against both visible and invisible enemies. Their spirits—angels, saints, and the honored dead—were woven into every aspect of life.

These people sought their ancestors in dreams, visited their graves, and called upon them for guidance. They understood the spirit world to be vast, filled with beings both benevolent and malevolent, and they used whatever means were available to them to navigate it and survive. This is why, in the case of Italian folk magic, the sacred and the profane exist side by side without contradiction. The sacred—prayers, iconography, Catholic rituals—merged seamlessly with the profane—pre-Christian spirits, gods, rites, and superstitions. There was no conflict, only necessity. Survival demanded both. Since folk magic is centered around connecting to the spirit world, it follows that this is a powerful way to connect with our ancestors. By connecting with our ancestors, we also connect to our cultural roots. Alternatively, we can say that researching our cultural roots is a path to connecting with our ancestors.

While discussing Italian folk magic, I want to share a common practice that I've adapted by removing the Catholic elements to show how these rituals can be customized to fit different belief systems. I also break them down to explain why they are effective.

Ritual to Dispel the Evil Eye

The malocchio (evil eye) is the belief that a gaze filled with envy, anger, or ill intent can bring misfortune to the person being looked at. It is one of the clearest examples of thought forms combined with strong emotions affecting people and their environment.

The most well-known method among Italians, both in Italy and throughout the diaspora, for diagnosing and curing the evil eye involves a bowl of water and drops of olive oil. Every practitioner has their own way of performing this ritual. There is no single "right" way—only what is effective and what is not. If a method is effective, it consistently produces the intended result.

Here's how the ritual is typically done:

1. The healer dips the index, middle, and ring fingers of their left hand into a small bowl of olive oil.
2. They allow at least three drops of oil to fall into a bowl of water.
3. The behavior of the oil in the water reveals whether the evil eye is present:

    » If the drops of oil stay separate from each other and the water, remaining static, this is a negative diagnosis. The evil eye *is not* present.

    » If the oil spreads, smears, or appears to dissolve into the water, this is a positive diagnosis. The evil eye *is* present.

    » If the oil drops pop and multiply, this also confirms the presence of the evil eye.

Once the evil eye is detected, the practitioner calls upon their protective spirits. Experienced practitioners will invoke spirits they already have a relationship with. If you are new to this practice, it's important to research protective spirits that resonate with you.

To remove the evil eye, follow these steps:

1. Take two sewing needles.

2. Insert the point of one into the eye of the other.

3. While doing this, recite the following incantation:

Incantation to Break the Evil Eye

Envy and evil eye,
Pierced and torn, they wither and die.
Shattered, scattered, their power reversed.
In the name of [*protective spirit(s) you invoke*],
Be gone, evil eye—dispersed!

The needles represent the act of severing the influence of the evil eye and piercing through negative energy. Like many folk magic rituals, this one is effective not just because of its physical elements but also because of the practitioner's intent, focus, and the connection they have with the unseen forces they invoke.

This is the point where you need a countdown to symbolize the evil eye weakening and losing its power. A common method in Italian folk magic is to use the days of the Christian Holy Week as a countdown. Another widely used approach is a nursery-rhyme-style countdown, both of which I'll include here:

Holy Week Countdown

Holy Monday, Holy Tuesday, Holy Wednesday, Holy Thursday, Holy Friday, Holy Saturday, Easter Sunday.

Alternatively, I like this countdown:

Nursery-Rhyme-Style Countdown

Once upon a time, there were seven brothers,
Who all caught the plague and died.
From seven, there were six.
From six, there were five.
From five, there were four.
From four, there were three.
From three, there were two.
From two, there was one.
And then—there were none.
In the name of [*insert protective spirit*],
The vile eye bursts and is dispersed!

4. Cross the water with the needle tips: Dip the points of the needles into the water three times, crossing them over the surface.

5. Sprinkle salt: Add three pinches of salt into the water.

6. Jab scissors into the water: Insert the scissors into the water three times, cutting through the water and oil each time.

7. Cut the air above the bowl: Hold the scissors above the bowl and cut through the air three times, symbolically breaking the energy link.

8. Dispose of the contents of the bowl: Once the spell is broken, take the contents of the bowl (water and oil) and pour it onto the ground where nothing will be harmed by the tiny amount of salt. Alternatively, you can pour it down the sink drain or flush it down the toilet. Some practitioners prefer to toss it in the trash, which also works.

    This method effectively removes the negative energy, breaking the influence of the evil eye.

To complete the ritual, do the following:

9. Draw the sign of protection and anoint: Dip your index finger into holy water (from a sacred site or charged with protective intentions) or holy oil (anointing oil created for protection). Using your finger, draw the sign of the cross three times over the person (or yourself, if they are not present). Alternatively, you may choose another protective symbol, such as the Elder Futhark rune Algiz (for protection), the Star of David, the pentagram, or the planetary symbol for Jupiter. While drawing these symbols, anoint the person's forehead and nape of the neck, sealing their protection and the ritual itself.

10. Close the ritual with gratitude: Finally, give thanks to your protective spirit(s), deity(ies), or any other beings you invoked during the ritual. Acknowledge their assistance and ask for their continued protection, both for the person you have cured and for yourself. Request that their blessings remain with you, keeping you both safe from harm and free from any negative influence, including the evil eye or malicious energy.

This closing ensures the ritual is sealed with gratitude and strengthens the bond between you and the protective forces you've invoked, leaving the subject shielded and the energy balanced.

Let's break down why this ritual works.

What Is the Evil Eye?

In short, the evil eye is an energetic or psychic attack. It is the result of someone—intentionally or unintentionally—projecting negative energy, jealousy, or ill intentions toward another person. This energetic projection can create an imbalance in the affected person's life, causing various symptoms or disturbances.

How Does the Evil Eye Manifest?

The evil eye can show up in a variety of ways, both physically and emotionally. Here are some common manifestations:

1. Physical Symptoms:
   » Headaches, especially behind the eyes.
   » Shortness of breath or chest pain, particularly in otherwise healthy individuals.
   » Anxiety, feelings of despair, or a pervasive sense of impending doom without any clear cause.
   » Accident-prone behavior. The afflicted person may experience more frequent accidents, especially when things seem fine on the surface.
   » Body aches. These are particularly common in healers or those who practice protective magic. These people often experience generalized pain with no apparent physical cause. This scenario can be likened to the aura acting as a shield—like a Kevlar vest that stops direct attacks but still transmits the kinetic force of those energetic hits, causing discomfort in the body.

2. Emotional and Psychological Symptoms:
   » The affected person may feel inexplicably out of sorts, as if their emotional or mental state is under constant strain.
   » Discord in relationships may appear as frequent misunderstandings or arguments that lead to emotional rifts, even in normally harmonious relationships.

3. Environmental Manifestations:
   » Objects or systems—like appliances, cars, or electronics—seem to fail all at once, creating an overwhelming sense of misfortune that doesn't seem to have any logical explanation.

- » There can be a general discordance or interference in everyday life, where things just feel "off" or seem to spiral beyond normal problems.

4. Pain in All Forms:
   - » The pain caused by the evil eye isn't just physical. It can be a combination of physical, mental, psychological, emotional, and spiritual pain. It is deeply subjective, as different people will feel and experience it differently.

5. Misfortune:
   - » This manifestation can range from a little bit of bad luck to extreme misfortune affecting all aspects of life, health, relationships, jobs, etc.
   - » When a person comes to me suspecting they have the evil eye, I listen closely to their symptoms. Whether it's a physical pain, a mental block, or an emotional struggle, I believe them because I have seen how these manifestations happen in real life. The evil eye isn't just some myth or superstition; it has tangible, real effects on a person's well-being.

The key to addressing the evil eye is understanding how energy flows and how we can protect ourselves and others from these energetic attacks.

As a healer, I can perceive the disruptive energy around a person, even from a distance. It's a sensation so familiar that as soon as they describe what's going on, I can feel it's not theirs. My body begins to register the telltale signs of spiritual illness, letting me know this energy is out of place. I don't need the traditional bowl of water and olive oil to confirm what both the afflicted person and I already sense.

Sometimes, however, it's not practical to use these tools, and in those cases, I can still proceed without them. That said, I always accommodate those who seek diagnostic confirmation, and I perform the ritual traditionally from time to time to keep my skills sharp.

But in my view, skipping the water and oil diagnosis doesn't harm the process. If malocchio (the evil eye) is present, the cure will remove it. If it isn't, the ritual still works as a cleansing, banishing, and protection process that benefits the person anyway.

So why does this ritual work? The concept of the evil eye is ancient and widely recognized. Diagnosis, in whatever form, helps identify the symptoms commonly associated with the evil eye. Once the affliction is named, it loses some of its power, making it easier to address. The behavior of the oil in the water confirms the malevolent presence, which is then contained in the bowl. The cure eliminates it, and the bowl's contents are disposed of.

In summary, the principles are simple: identify, contain, destroy, dispose, and refresh protection.

In my culture, any form of psychic attack is labeled malocchio and dealt with in the same way. I don't reinvent the wheel when my ancestors' methods work just fine, so I follow their lead. When handling any psychic attack, I apply the same principles as I do for removing the evil eye: call on my protective spirits, diagnose/identify, capture/contain, disarm/destroy, dispose, and finally, reinforce protection.

Today, I feel that malocchio and the knowledge of how to dispel it are as relevant as ever. Social media is an incredible tool for connecting with distant family and friends, finding communities of like-minded people, and even marketing goods and services. However, it is also a breeding ground for rampant envy and jealousy. Not all of it is malicious or intentional, but when someone shares their seemingly perfect life online, thousands of people—friends, family, even strangers—are watching. Many of them experience feelings of comparison, insecurity, imposter syndrome, and envy.

These feelings are true even among those who love and care for us. And it's not just the people who are genuinely envious; it's also those who pretend to be our friends while secretly wishing us failure or misfortune. Sadly, not everyone has our best interests at heart. I've seen firsthand how envy on social media can manifest in striking ways. Someone posts about their "perfect" life—whether real or exaggerated—and the comments are filled with admiration, as well as hidden (or not-so-hidden) feelings of inferiority from others. Then, out of nowhere, the seemingly perfect life turns into a public disaster, as if misfortune strikes just to prove that appearances aren't everything.

We've already touched on this, but it bears repeating: To guard against the evil eye, we return to an old truth. William Shakespeare said it well, "Have more than you show, speak less than you know." My elders always taught me to maintain humility and avoid boasting, as this only invites envy and makes us a target for the evil eye. This advice doesn't apply just to material possessions but also to knowledge, skills, and even health. For example, if someone is blessed with good looks or perfect health, it's important not to flaunt these things, especially in the presence of those who may envy them.

I've noticed an interesting phenomenon regarding envy, particularly with physical appearance. One case that often stands out is when someone with thick, healthy, and long hair receives constant compliments. It almost seems as though the more they are praised for their hair, the more they start to feel dissatisfied with it. Suddenly, they book a hair appointment, as if triggered by the compliments, and the results are almost always disastrous. The beautiful hair is drastically altered, sometimes to the point where it looks unrecognizable. The color ruined, texture changed, and the hair that once turned heads is no longer the lustrous mane it once was. This phenomenon has always baffled me. After years of experiencing this firsthand and hearing similar stories from friends, I began to wonder if something other than mere coincidence was at play. With so much magic and lore surrounding hair, it's hard not to consider the possibility that unseen forces might be involved.

The following is another common tradition in Italian folk magic that is easily adapted to any practice.

Summer Solstice Water (Saint John's Water)

Saint John's water is an ancient tradition tied to both food and ritual, religion and magic, with roots deeply intertwined in the feast of San Giovanni Battista (Saint John the Baptist). This ritual has been passed down for generations, serving as both remedy and sacred preparation, long before modern medicine emerged.

The night of June 23 to 24, known as Saint John's Eve or Midsummer's Eve, is one of the most magical nights of the year. It aligns with the summer solstice, when the sun reaches its peak. This energy is said to charge the water prepared on this night, capturing the powerful essence of the summer solstice, which occurs between June 20 and 22 in the northern hemisphere and December 20 to 23 in the southern hemisphere.

In addition to the solstice, this time is also linked to Saint Anastasia, whose feast day is on December 22 (Greek Orthodox) or December 25 (Catholic). She is known for her powers over potions and curses, and is invoked to break hexes and curses, offering spiritual protection.

Whether in the northern or southern hemisphere, the plants gathered during the solstice are filled with potent energy. The sun, plants, dew, and night air combine to amplify their protective powers. Saint John's water was believed to ward off evil spirits, misfortune, and even prevent droughts or storms that could harm crops.

The ritual is a way of absorbing nature's maximum energy, from nascent fruits to wild herbs and morning dew, all of which were thought to have miraculous properties.

Herbs for Saint John's Water

Traditionally, various herbs are used in the preparation for Saint John's water, including

- » Lavender
- » Wild fennel
- » Mallow
- » Wormwood
- » Verbena
- » Rosemary
- » Poppy
- » Rose
- » Mint
- » Chamomile

- » Passionflower
- » Elderberry
- » Sage
- » Saint John's wort (considered especially effective against the evil eye)

Saint John's wort, known as the "devil-chasing herb," is the most potent in dispelling negative energies. Other herbs like sage, mint, and mugwort also carry protective qualities. Many people dry these herbs to create teas for year-round use or prepare traditional Saint John's herb ravioli, a special dish for the feast day on June 24, particularly popular in Emilia and the province of Parma, where the tradition continues today.

Nocino, Snails, and Summer Solstice Water: Italian Customs

1. Nocino Liqueur

An Italian tradition involves picking unripe walnuts with their husks during the night, an act performed only by women. These walnuts are then placed in 95 percent food-grade alcohol to macerate for at least thirty days. It is then filtered and bottled. The resulting nocino liqueur is consumed no earlier than November 1 in the northern hemisphere (All Saints' Day). If you have access to picking unripe walnuts in the southern hemisphere, you will follow the same procedure. The only difference is the resulting nocino is consumed no earlier than May 1.

2. Snails and the Miraculous Dew

In Rome, particularly in families deeply connected to tradition, snails are gathered on Saint John's Eve (June 23), much like herbs. They are believed to benefit from the "miraculous dew" collected during the night. Afterward, they're cooked in a tomato sauce.

The snails are considered a good omen not just because of the dew but also because of their horns (antennae)—resembling those of the devil.

Eating them is thought to chase away evil, though personally, I find the reasoning a bit confusing. Eating snails because they have horns like the devil seems more like inviting in the devil than keeping him away. I don't partake in this tradition, as I consider snails my friends. Cooking them is a whole process, and one I can't stomach. It starts with purging them for a week (starving them) before cooking them alive. Enough said on that.

3. Summer Solstice Water (Saint John's Water or Saint Anastasia's Water)

Now, here's how you make summer solstice water, also called Saint John's water (or what I would call Saint Anastasia's water for my friends in the southern hemisphere):

1. Harvesting: After sunset on June 23 (or the summer solstice), gather the flowers and herbs that are in season and available to you, choosing them ethically.

2. Infusion: Place the plants in a basin with spring or well water and leave it outside overnight, so it absorbs the dew.

3. Morning Use: On the morning of June 24, use the water to wash your hands and face while saying morning prayers for blessings and protection.

4. Leftover Water: Don't throw away the unused water. It can be given to a friend as a gift, but be sure to use it up quickly because it spoils.

What's Going On Here?

This ritual is all about harvesting plants when the sun is at its peak, infusing them in water, and letting that water absorb the night air and dew. Magic, as always, comes with a cost. Once the plants are cut, they release their life force and begin to die. Their essence gets infused in the water, which is then charged by the night air and dew. The result is a potion containing the plant spirits.

Is Saint John's Water Magical Only on June 23?

Traditionally, Saint John's water is made on June 23, but if you don't subscribe to that specific worldview, you can make it by harvesting plants the night before the summer solstice. The resulting water will be summer solstice water. You can also use the same technique at any time of the year to craft potions, adapting the plants and seasonal energies as needed.

Saint Peter's Sailboat: Divination by Egg White in Water

Oomancy is divination using eggs, and one common method is interpreting the shape formed when raw egg whites are dropped into hot water. This practice resembles ceromancy, the divination of shapes formed by melted wax in water.

Saint Peter's Sailboat is an Italian folk tradition with roots in northern Italy. This ritual, tied to the cult of Saint Peter, dates back to the 8th century and is performed on the night of June 28 to coincide with the feast of Saints Peter and Paul. Initially used to predict weather conditions vital for farming, the ritual has expanded to include family fortunes and blessings. In the southern hemisphere, this weather divination ritual would take place on December 28, to coincide with it being a week after summer solstice. My relatives located in the southern hemisphere still refer to it as Saint Peter's Sailboat because they brought this tradition with them to the southern hemisphere when they immigrated from Italy.

How to Make Saint Peter's Sailboat

1. Prepare the Water: On the evening of June 28 (or December 28), fill a transparent vase or carafe with cold water.
2. Add the Egg White: Gently pour just the egg white into the water.

3. Leave Outdoors: Place the container outside overnight—ideally in the garden, under a tree, or on a windowsill—to allow the dew and fresh air to interact with it.

4. Morning Interpretation: The following morning, the egg white will crystallize into filamentous shapes resembling boat sails.

How to Interpret the Sailboat

- » Open sails: Predicts sunny weather and good fortune for the year.
- » Closed, thin sails: Forecasts rain or bad weather.

People often ask Saint Peter a question about their family's future or well-being while pouring the egg white.

- » Tall, open sails are seen as a sign of an upcoming wedding or birth.

Asking about a business's success would be interpreted by the shape:

- » Open sails: Yes.
- » Closed, thin sails: No.

The egg white slowly dissolves by midday, completing the process.

Why Does the Boat Form?

Folk belief attributes the shape to Saint Peter, the fisherman and ferryman of souls, who is said to blow into the water to show his closeness to the faithful. Scientifically, the phenomenon results from the temperature difference between night and day. The evening's humidity causes the egg white to coagulate, and the heat rising from the ground or windowsill carries it up, forming the sailboat shape.

The Magical Mechanism

Saint Peter's sailboat is a form of weather divination, an ancient practice where weather patterns are believed to predict the outcome of earthly matters. By observing the natural world—weather, wildlife, and seasonal changes—we can interpret the unseen forces at work around us, just as our ancestors did.

Personal Connection

Weather, as a divination tool, plays a central role in daily life in Italy and among Italian communities worldwide. Conversations often begin with a weather report and its personal significance (such as health, mood, or agricultural conditions). Similarly, fellow witches of all cultural backgrounds often discuss the weather and its symbolic meaning, reinforcing the idea that we are constantly interacting with both the seen and unseen worlds.

Adaptation to Your Practice

Understanding the principles behind these rituals allows you to adapt them to your own magical practice. Explore your own culture or a tradition that inspires you and make it your own. Divination is about connecting with the world around us, interpreting signs, and adjusting our practices accordingly.

Tools of the Craft

Before we explore the tools of folk magic, let me say this: You don't need anything fancy to get started. The heart of this practice isn't in what you own—it's in what you know, what you carry, and how you show up. Everything you need is either already within you or readily available in your surroundings. Folk magic is the magic of the people. It's deeply rooted in a connection to nature and the spirit world. The power lies within you, and the world around you offers everything you need to work your magic.

The Elements as Tools in Folk Magic

Air: In folk magic, air is a tool for connection and communication. It represents breath, sound, and the unseen forces that carry energy. When we direct our breath or the flow of air, we activate spells or send messages to the spirit world. Air is also a purifier. Simply opening a window to let in fresh air clears out stale energy. But my ancestors were wary of strong winds, believing they carried demonic spirits that could enter through an open mouth. Whether or not you believe in that, the force of wind can be unsettling, and I use its power to clear negative energy by burning incense, letting the air carry it away. Air's true power in folk magic is its ability to carry energy, messages, and offerings to the unseen world.

Fire: Fire is a tool of transformation in folk magic, symbolizing purification, change, and the release of energy. We use fire to cleanse tools, cook food, and invoke spirits. Light a candle or burn incense, and you're sending offerings to the spirits, releasing energy into the universe. Fire can also break down objects, freeing their energy, but you've got to be careful. Burning something with harmful energy will release that energy and cause trouble. In pyromancy, we read the flames to gain insight from the spirit world. Fire's power lies in its dual nature as both creator and destroyer, making it essential in folk magic for transformation and invocation.

Water: Water is sacred in folk magic—our tool for cleansing, blessing, and healing. It's a vessel for energy—charged by moonlight, or sacred sites, or infused with plants for specific purposes. Water can create protective potions, heal, or even curse, depending on our intent. It's used for divination too, as we scry its reflective surface to reveal visions or messages. Water channels energy from the divine and the spirit world, making it a versatile tool. Its ability to nourish life while adapting to its surroundings makes it both soothing and powerful.

Earth: Earth is our grounding tool in folk magic, representing stability, fertility, and security. Earth is where we root ourselves; it's the foundation of life. In folk magic, we use earth for protection and manifestation, whether by creating effigies, burying objects for safekeeping, or using sacred dirt for blessings. Earth holds energy, and we can tap into it to manifest our desires or protect ourselves from harm. Grounding practices, like standing barefoot on the earth or burying something for protection, restore balance. Earth offers support, nourishment, and protection. It's the foundation of all magical work.

Balancing the Elements: In folk magic, the key is balance. When one element feels off, we use the others to temper it. Take, for example, someone who's overthinking, stuck in their head. To bring them back into balance, earthy activities like walking barefoot or eating grounding foods can help. The elements work together, each bringing its unique energy to heal, protect, and transform. Once you understand how to work with the elements, you can shape your world and your magic.

Useful Objects in Folk Magic

Whether you're new to this practice or have been working with it for years, this list of useful objects is meant to inspire you. I've been practicing for a long time, and I still feel excited when I see the tools others use. These are the items I use in my own practice. Some I use daily, others only on occasion. These are all things you likely already have in your home, or they can be easily obtained free from friends and family or purchased inexpensively at secondhand shops. This is not an exhaustive list, and it doesn't represent every folk witch's tools, but these are what work for me:

> **Broom:** The broom is a cleansing tool, plain and simple. I use it to sweep out stagnant energy, to clear a space before ritual. As a symbol of spirit flight, the broom marks the threshold between sacred and ordinary.

Lighter and safety matches: Self-explanatory, but I'll add that I use a match instead of a candle when I need to quickly invoke a spirit or when time is short.

Heatproof surface: I use a large ceramic tile left over from a floor installation. Since my practice often involves fire, it protects the surface I'm working on.

Large pot with a lid: Or a cauldron. I repurposed an old stainless steel pot to use as a mixing bowl, for heating over a flame, collecting rainwater, and safely burning things. The lid is crucial for safety; it helps smother flames or contain too much smoke.

Small pot with a lid: I have a little cast-iron cauldron for holding the charred remains of incense. I use it for fire safety, and the charred remains often go into spells or into black salt.

Candleholders: I use glass candleholders that fit the candles I regularly use. I prefer jar-type holders with an open top, like hurricane candleholders, and reuse them repeatedly. I personalize these jars by gluing printed images onto them. The images come off easily with water when no longer needed.

Incense holder/burner: I use different holders depending on the incense. For stick incense, I have a clay bowl with salt (now mixed with years of incense ash). For resin, I use a burner with a tealight underneath to toast the incense slowly. I also have a wooden incense holder for sticks.

Oil/wax warmer: I prefer ceramic, but these warmers come in various materials and styles, including heated by a tea light, battery-operated, or electric. I use one for warming wax infused with herbs, oils, and resins for magical purposes.

Tin foil: Tin foil is incredibly versatile in my practice. I use it to line pots, wax warmers, or incense burners. It also helps me create premeasured herb packets, cover open containers, and make figures or talismans. Its reflective properties are great for protection spells.

Mortar and pestle: I have a stone mortar and pestle dedicated to magical work. It's used for grinding resins and herbs into fine powders to release their oils and create stronger incense blends.

Spoon: I use a small coffee spoon to measure ingredients.

Paintbrush: A small, stiff paintbrush is helpful for sweeping out the contents of my mortar.

Bowl: I use one for mixing ingredients and holding water.

Empty jars and bottles: These are used for storing ingredients or used as candleholders.

Funnel: A funnel is useful for transferring oils between bottles.

Strainer: A strainer is useful for straining herbs and resins after they've been infused in oils. I prefer using nylon stockings (a neat trick my friend taught me), as they don't absorb the oils like cheesecloth or coffee filters.

Twine, cotton string, cotton thread, yarn: They are used for knot magic, binding spells, protection amulets, tying herb bundles, and crafting magical items. Red natural-fiber yarn is used in many traditions and is especially useful for protection and binding spells.

Box: Boxes are for keeping things contained—spells, charms, intentions. I use them to hold magical workings that need time to settle or stay hidden. A closed box is a sealed spell. A plain box can be used for storing items away from prying eyes.

Notebook and pen: I always carry a small notebook to record ideas, omens, or anything related to my craft.

Journal or diary: I keep several journals for different aspects of my practice, like a commonplace book, grimoires, a book of shrines, and a dream journal. I'll go into more detail about these in a later chapter.

Deck of playing cards: The cards are used for cartomancy and spirit communication. Cards help predict the future, offer guidance before casting a spell, or check the outcome of a spell.

Pendulum: I use this for yes/no answers when communicating with spirits.

Scissors/knife: Scissors and knives are both tools and amulets of protection. They help ward against curses and are used in hex-breaking rituals. As tools, they're great for cutting string or harvesting plants. As amulets, they protect from the evil eye and remove unwanted energies.

Iron: Items made of iron, like a cast-iron cauldron, door knocker, or nails, are believed to protect against malefic spirits and energies.

Mirror: I use mirrors to send harm back, scry for hidden truths or spirit messages, and shield against the evil eye. After some workings, I cover the mirror to close it. To lock it, I place it face-down or wrap it in black, white, or red cloth—sometimes with a protective sign or a spoken charm to seal it until it's needed again.

Religious iconography: I use religious iconography as tools of devotion and protection—objects that carry both faith and power. These aren't just symbols, they're helpers. I place them on my altar, carry them for safety, or use them in workings when I need strength beyond my own. They connect me to something older, deeper, and remind me I'm never working alone.

Rosary/prayer beads: I use rosary or prayer beads as both a devotional and magical tool. They help me focus during prayers, protect against harm, and anchor my intentions. Sometimes I recite traditional prayers; other times, I weave in charms or blessings, bead by bead, like a spell whispered through rhythm and breath.

Jewelry: I use jewelry in folk magic the way others might use amulets or talismans. Each piece I wear has a purpose—protection, attraction, remembrance. Some are inherited, carrying the spirit of those who wore them before me. Others are charged with prayer, anointed with magical oil, or programmed with a specific purpose. Rings, necklaces, earrings—they're not just adornment, they're tools woven into daily life. Secret spells worn on the body.

Clothing and accessories: I use head coverings and specific clothing as tools in folk magic to mark sacred intent, protect my energy, and signal to spirits that I'm entering ritual space. A scarf or shawl over my head helps me focus, shields me from unwanted influence, and connects me to the lineage of women before me who did the same. Certain colors, fabrics, or garments hold memory and meaning—turning everyday wear into quiet acts of devotion and power.

Perfume and makeup: Perfume and makeup are part of my magic too. Scents carry memory, spirit, and intention—what I wear depends on what I need. Some perfumes connect me to my ancestors, some are for protection, others draw something in. Makeup is a kind of sigil work for me: color, shape, placement—each stroke can carry meaning. These aren't just for appearance; they're spells I wear on my skin.

These are the tools that work for me, and they might inspire you to find or repurpose your own magical tools. What's important is how you connect with them and how they support your practice.

Some Staples in a Folk Witch's Cupboard

Candles: I keep two types of candles. First are the basic paraffin tea lights, which I use for heat and lighting. The second type is spell candles, made with specific ingredients for specific purposes, and these are burned only for their intended magic. These can be purchased or made by the practitioner.

Incense: Incense comes in several forms: sticks, cones, and resin chunks like myrrh, copal, and styrax. There are also incense powders and loose incense blends, which can be bought or crafted by the practitioner.

Plants: I store edible herbs in my kitchen pantry and herbs unsafe for consumption in a secure, clearly labeled cabinet. When my children were small, I didn't keep anything unsafe in the house. Folk witches develop strong, personal relationships with a select group of plant spirits, and as we grow in experience, our herb supplies tend to shrink, becoming more intentional and meaningful. Folk magic is deeply connected to the land, and we primarily use plants grown locally, whether cultivated in a garden or foraged from the wild. We have a responsibility to the land—to take only what we need and to support the growth of cultivated plants without disturbing the wild ones.

Salt: If I could have only one ingredient, salt would be it. Fortunately, I don't have to choose. Salt is incredibly versatile: It cleanses, banishes malignant energy, and protects. It can be used alone or in water, to bless, to form protective boundaries, or to clear energy from objects. A common practice is burying objects in salt to remove any attached negative energy. Be cautious, though, not to bury anything that could be damaged. Salt can be carried as a protective amulet or used for a "freezing" spell in place of a freezer (like when you need to keep something sealed or trapped but don't want others to know). It's portable, easy to get, and has endless magical uses. I always carry a small packet from a restaurant or an airtight container of coarse sea salt in my bag. Salt's properties align closely with its physical qualities: Sea salt carries the energy of the ocean, and table salt embodies the energy of the earth. It draws moisture from everything it touches, making it antibacterial and a natural preservative. It's truly an all-purpose tool.

Honey: Honey is used in spells to sweeten things up. It's sticky, sweet, golden, and full of the essence of the flowers from which the bees gather nectar. Honey doesn't spoil, and its antibacterial properties translate well to magic. It's a highly versatile ingredient, used in love, beauty, health, and even death spells. Historically, honey has been offered to deities and spirits, carrying with it blessings and sweetness.

Dirt: Graveyard dirt and churchyard dirt (dirt or soil from any sacred site, really) are prized in folk magic for their sacred qualities. These soils absorb the energies of years, even centuries, of emotions, prayers, and blessings. I prefer graveyard dirt, or more often, small stones from graves, because they're portable and versatile. Graveyard dirt carries the full spectrum of human emotions—from deep sorrow to the joy of release—and is filled with the spirits of the dead, as well as the living energy of the land. It's a potent tool in both protective and baneful magic, making it a powerful addition to any witch's practice.

There are a number of ways to collect graveyard dirt respectfully. This is how I do it. You are welcome to do it this way or some other way. Introduce yourself and announce your intention at the gate of the cemetery. Ask the spirits to grant you safe passage. If you get a bad feeling, that's a no. Leave and come back another time. Otherwise, proceed. Choose a spot that is not a specific grave. You may have to dig a little with a spoon to get down to plain dirt without grass or roots. If you need a stone, take the smallest one you need for your purpose. Cover the spot you dug up and place your payment/offering on the same spot. The offerings we left were tobacco, coins, and an act of service in the form of cleaning up an old grave or picking up trash. On the way out, thank the spirits and respectfully tell them they are not welcome to follow you.

Let's break it down:

1. Introduce yourself to the spirits and announce your intention.
2. Ask for permission and their protection.
3. Take only what you need.
4. Leave the area better than you found it.
5. Give an offering or payment.
6. Thank the spirits and bid farewell and be clear that you do not permit them to follow you.

I also apply steps 1 to 5 to foraging in nature.

Items Foraged from Nature

The use of natural items like dirt, twigs, branches, leaves, seeds, stones, thorns, feathers, reptile skin sheds, and animal remains has been a staple in folk magic for as long as the practice has existed. These items are especially important for those who work closely with land spirits. As with graveyard dirt, it's essential to approach foraging with respect and care. Tread lightly, for land spirits are powerful forces that should not be taken lightly. Always make sure you're following local laws and guidelines when gathering these items. Respect for nature and the spirits that reside there is key to maintaining a harmonious and safe practice.

Waters: Waters play an essential role in folk magic, with countless types and uses found across cultures. These include perfumed waters, colognes, water from sacred sites, moon water, floor washes, holy water, and war water. Each type serves a specific purpose, whether it's for cleansing, banishing, blessing, or even hexing. The power of water in folk magic is versatile, and it can be charged with intention to serve a wide array of magical needs.

Oils: Anointing oils are deeply rooted in religious and spiritual practices across cultures, and their use is integral to folk magic. The tactile and fragrant nature of oils connects us to ancient traditions. My favorite oils are those I create by adding compatible plants and resins to a carrier oil, allowing them to infuse over time in a dark cupboard. Oils are widely available, and many practitioners prefer natural oils and blends. However, essential oils require extreme care, as they can be harmful to pregnant or lactating women, babies, and pets. Personally, I use both natural and synthetic oils with great results. Oils are used for blessing, anointing the body and objects, and imbuing them with the magical properties of the ingredients infused within.

Garlic: Garlic holds a special place in folk magic, especially when it comes to hex-breaking and protection. According to my Italian ancestors, garlic is literally Saint Michael the Archangel—a belief passed down through generations. This belief stems from garlic's remarkable ability to cast out and repel evil spirits. Beyond its magical uses, raw garlic is known for its antiviral, antibacterial, and anti-inflammatory properties, making it a powerful remedy both externally and internally.

Garlic always brings to mind the late Dr. Leo Buscaglia, who shared a story from his childhood. His Italian mother, always looking out for him, would send him to school wearing and reeking of garlic. It wasn't just for flavor; it was to protect him from illness, as they believed, the evil eye.

Garlic can be used in many ways in folk magic: It can be ingested, worn as an amulet, or used in spells to benefit from its protective and hex-breaking properties. Whether it's hanging in a doorway, added to a protective charm, or included in a cleansing ritual, garlic remains one of the most reliable guardians against malevolent forces.

Onion: Onions, with their many layers, have long been associated with uncovering what is hidden or concealed. The act of peeling away each layer mirrors the process of revealing secrets, exposing the truth, or unraveling deceit. In folk magic, onions are often used in spells designed to uncover hidden motives, expose enemies, or bring lies to the surface.

Onions also have a place in love magic. The layers can symbolize the unfolding of love or the removal of barriers to emotional connection. They're often included in spells to help break down walls between people, allowing for deeper intimacy and understanding. Whether used to expose an enemy's ill intentions or to open the heart in love, the onion's layers offer a powerful symbolic tool for peeling back the layers of life and revealing what's beneath.

Once we understand what a folk witch does, it's just as important to know how we do it—through the tools we keep, the ingredients we gather, and the ways we care for and work with them over time.

Arts and Crafts

When I was little, my mother embroidered my clothing with red thread for protection. I can still picture the ladybug stitched on my pajamas, my initials carefully monogrammed on a cardigan, or just a few quick stitches of red thread hidden in a garment. Red stitching was her quiet, loving way of imbuing my clothing with a layer of protection. Handmade crocheted blankets and knitted booties were also part of our family's apotropaic essentials, offering warmth not only to the body but to the spirit as well.

When I first started on my path, I bought things like amulets and magical tools. I still treasure a few of those early purchases; they hold sentimental value and carry memories of the journey I've taken. But over time, I have found myself leaning more and more toward creating my own magical items. There's something deeply personal and empowering about making things by hand, infusing them with your own energy and intentions. I was fortunate to learn skills like hand sewing, embroidery, and crochet at a young age, and now, these crafts are an integral part of my practice. If I need to make something that requires a skill I haven't yet mastered, I simply turn to the Internet for a how-to video. The beauty of this path is that the possibilities are endless, and whether through knitting, sewing, or any other craft, you can weave your magic into the very fabric of what you create. It's a deeply fulfilling and personal way to connect with the spiritual world.

Reuse and Recycle

I was raised by immigrant parents who came to North America with nothing. They worked tirelessly, sacrificing so much so that their children could have opportunities they never had. From them, I learned the value of not wasting anything: Use what you have, mend what is broken, and if something can't be repaired, salvage the parts that are still functional and find new ways to reuse them.

My parents primarily bought secondhand when they could and saved up for the things that truly needed to be purchased new. That's where my love of tag sales, rummage sales, bazaars, and thrift stores comes from. I have fond memories of going through stacks of items, searching for hidden gems, and feeling a deep connection to the resourcefulness my parents instilled in me. I can still hear their voices in my head as I sift through the treasures at a thrift shop, reminding me that the best things are often the ones that have been lovingly used and are waiting to find a new purpose.

This mindset didn't just shape how I live day to day; it's woven into my magical practice as well. I reuse objects when I can—whether it's repurposing the same candleholder, using a glass jar over and over, or recycling old offerings for a new spell. I find great power in using items that have already served a purpose and are still full of energy. And just like with my everyday life, I don't waste in my magic. When a working has proven effective, I recycle it, adapting and tweaking it as needed, rather than discarding it. To me, there's something deeply powerful about reusing, recycling, and honoring the resources we already have—in both the mundane and the magical realms. It's a practice rooted in gratitude, sustainability, and respect for the energy that surrounds us.

You Cast a Spell, so Now What?

Now that you've cast a spell, how do you know it worked? Sometimes, the answer is simple: You just know. There's a subtle shift in the energy around you, like the air changing from stillness to a soft breeze, or vice versa. It's a quiet feeling, almost like the world around you has paused for a moment to acknowledge what you've just set in motion. But that isn't always the case. Sometimes the signs are more overt, and the proof shows up physically, either within the working itself or in the form of an omen in your environment that you can read as confirmation. As you gain experience, your ability to feel and interpret these shifts becomes more attuned. You begin to recognize the signs and symbols of magic more clearly, as if the universe itself is speaking to you through your senses.

In candle magic, for example, the way a candle burns can be a clear indicator of how your working is progressing. A candle that burns cleanly and effortlessly without excessive dripping or black smoke is a good sign. This usually indicates that the spell has been well received and is moving forward smoothly. On the other hand, if the candle struggles to stay lit, emits black smoke, or deposits soot on the inside of a glass votive, that's a clear sign of interference or resistance. Something is blocking the flow of energy, or there's an obstacle in your way.

At this point in my practice, I can feel the energy shift around me, and I trust that my spirits are always right there with me, guiding and assisting. I never do a magical working without consulting my spirits first. For me, this always involves doing a tarot card reading to check in with the energy and the guidance I'm working with. I also do a tarot reading after the working to confirm whether it's gone according to plan. The cards help me tune in to the results and guide me in refining my approach if needed.

I also believe in the importance of monitoring and evaluating the results of any spell. If a working only partially manifests, I don't dismiss it as a failure. I pay attention to what *did* succeed and especially take note of any unintended consequences. These are usually where the lesson lies. Unintended outcomes often trace back to something I overlooked. Maybe I wasn't clear enough in my intention, or I failed to account for an important variable in the working. Each experience, whether a success or a lesson in disguise, adds to my practice, and I always make a note of what I can learn and adjust next time. It's this process of continual growth and awareness that strengthens my relationship with magic and my own intuitive abilities.

Discarding Spell Remains

The question I get most often about spell work is, "What do we do with the remains?" I believe that once a spell is complete and its energy has been spent, the physical ingredients no longer hold power and can usually be discarded in the trash, except for tools and objects intended for reuse. I cleanse these and put them away for the next time I need them. Some traditions recommend burying spell remains, but this doesn't always consider the potential harm to the environment. Proper disposal must be with respect for nature spirits and our ecological responsibility. Common disposal methods include burying remains for spells related to growth or protection, but only when using biodegradable materials that won't harm the soil or wildlife. I also recommend burying on your own property. When I lived in an apartment in an urban center, I buried the remains of spells—when safe to do so—in my potted plants. Flowing water, such as rivers, streams, or the ocean, can be used for cleansing or sending intentions outward, but only if the materials are natural and nonpolluting to avoid harming wildlife.

Burning is another method used to purify and release energy, ensuring the ashes are scattered safely. Trash disposal is ideal for banishing or letting go, and since I believe the energy is spent once the spell is complete, this is the method I use for almost all my spell remains. Flushing it away with water in a sink or toilet is an option for dissolvable, nontoxic substances used in cleansing or banishing work. Composting or feeding wildlife is possible when using safe, organic materials that contribute to nature rather than harm it. Some items, such as jars, tools, and crystals, can be cleansed and reused instead of discarded. Ultimately, the key is to dispose of spell remains in a way that aligns with your practice while being mindful of the natural world.

The Role of Divination in Folk Magic

I was raised in a world where divination wasn't just a practice; it was a way of life. Fortune-tellers, psychics, cartomancers—whatever name they went by—were not merely sought; they were revered. They were consulted as frequently as, if not more than, clergy. When I was just six years old and showed a glimmer of interest in playing with cards, my family encouraged me to learn how to read them. And so, I did. I've been reading cards ever since, always in awe of the power they hold to connect me to unseen forces.

In my family, the most common method of divination was dream interpretation. Dreams were a regular part of conversation, especially when someone was going through uncertain or difficult times. Every family had at least one member who was proficient at interpreting dreams, and those dream interpreters were deeply respected. Our dreams, we believed, held all the answers to our questions, and they were the place where we interacted with our beloved dead and other spirits who, on rare occasions, would send direct messages, but more often, we would need to interpret the symbols and messages carefully. It was in the dream realm that the answers were often veiled, requiring patience and understanding to decode.

Another significant form of divination that was woven into the fabric of my upbringing was the interpretation of omens. Omens were everywhere, and my family paid close attention to the signs that appeared in the world around us. Divination was not just something practiced occasionally; it was integrated into our daily life. It was how we communicated with the unseen world and how we stayed in contact with our spirits.

Divination is, and always will be, a vital part of my folk magic practice. It's how I navigate the complexities of life and keep my connection with the spirits strong. I am always observing my environment, interpreting the messages I receive through dreams, omens, and, especially, nature. Nature itself speaks in whispers if you know how to listen.

As I mentioned earlier, on a practical level, I rely heavily on card reading—specifically, tarot. I consult the cards before any magical workings to check if the time is right and if it's safe to proceed. Afterward, I use tarot to evaluate if the working was successful and what effects it has had. But divination isn't reserved for magical workings alone. Like my ancestors before me, I use tarot for much more: to aid in interpreting dreams, making decisions, understanding how situations will unfold, uncovering obstacles, and communicating with spirits. Over the decades—fifty years, to be exact—I've expanded my divination practice beyond the basics. I consult tarot to help me understand what has already occurred (reading the past). I ask tarot for guidance on goal setting, specifically: "What else can I do, in addition to what I am already doing, to achieve my goal?" I also use the cards for decision-making and to gain insight into myself and the world around me.

No matter what method of divination you use, the goal remains the same: to gain insight, to understand, and to navigate life with clarity. In the context of folk magic, divination is a compass that helps us make sense of the shifting tides of existence. It guides us, protects us, and helps us align with the forces of the universe. It is, quite simply, indispensable.

As we grow in our practice, we often find ourselves drawn to new methods of divination—some familiar, some foreign—and over time, we make them our own. We learn by watching, by doing, by listening to our spirits and trusting what resonates in our bones. Just like the folk witches before us, we shape our divination practices to fit the rhythm of our lives, our geography, our culture, weaving together tradition, intuition, and experience until they become second nature—a living, breathing part of our magic.

The Power of Specialization in Folk Magic

In folk magic, there's immense power in specialization. It's not about doing everything or trying to master every technique under the sun; it's about finding what works for you and honing it. Whether you're just beginning your journey or you've walked the path for years, experimentation is key. Try different practices, different spells, different rituals. Explore the vast landscape of magical tools and techniques.

But once you find something that resonates with you, something that works, don't move on too quickly. Stick with it. Building your magical practice is a lot like building muscle. The more you engage with something that works, the stronger your connection to that practice becomes. It's like a muscle memory, a rhythm that deepens over time. Repeating the same spell, ritual, or working helps to wear a groove—a familiar path that your energy naturally follows. This repetition makes it easier to access the energy you need, achieving your desired result with greater speed and less effort each time. The act of repetition isn't a sign of laziness or stagnation; it's an indication of power. When you repeat a practice, you're reinforcing your connection to it. You're carving deeper channels in your consciousness and energy field that make your magical work more efficient. The more you engage with what works, the more you build momentum, and that momentum fuels your practice, allowing you to see quicker results with less force.

Folk magic is rooted in the mundane as much as in the mystical. It's about creating an intimate relationship with your tools, with the land, with the elements. Repeating the same actions until they become second nature allows you to move through your practice with ease and flow, relying on the muscle of your magical experience to bring forth results that are both powerful and precise. Over time, that groove becomes a well-worn path, one that's effortless to walk and one that always leads to your desired outcome. This is where the magic becomes your own—personalized, refined, and potent. Don't be afraid to specialize, and don't hesitate to deepen your connection to the practices that resonate with you the most. The power of folk magic lies in your ability to build and refine your own practice, step by step, working with what you know best.

Critical Thinking in Folk Magic

Critical thinking is an essential tool in folk magic, not just for understanding the mechanics of your work but also for refining and evolving your practice. When you observe consistent results with a spell, you should analyze what worked, why it worked, and how it can be adapted for different circumstances. Magic isn't just about blindly following rituals; it's about working with what you have, adjusting as needed, and being results-oriented. I always take note of what spells consistently yield the results I need, and I don't hesitate to recycle them, modifying and tweaking them to suit the new situation at hand.

Magic isn't a one-size-fits-all practice. The beauty of folk magic lies in its adaptability. If a spell works, you use it repeatedly, but you also tweak it when different needs arise. For example, the Freeze Enemy spell I've mentioned several times has been effective for me because it's adaptable. It's a simple spell where you write the name or place the photo of someone who is threatening your peace and safety into a glass of water and place it in the freezer. As the water freezes around the paper or photo, it's as if the person is "frozen" in their actions, their behavior halted. But I've taken that basic concept—the "freezing" mechanism—and applied it to other situations that benefit from a pause, a cooling down, or a temporary halt. The subject doesn't have to be an antagonist; you can use this method for anything that needs to be subdued, cooled, or set aside for a time. For example, if you're dealing with overwhelming thoughts or emotions, freezing those thoughts in time can allow you space to regain your peace. If a situation or project is stagnating, freezing it in place might give you the clarity or time you need to strategize before taking action.

That's the core of critical thinking in folk magic—recognizing what works, analyzing why it works, and adapting it to suit the new goals or challenges. It's about being flexible, willing to adjust, and knowing when to apply a well-worn technique in new ways. This approach gives you both a deep understanding of your magical tools and a greater sense of mastery over your practice, allowing you to create practical solutions in a world that often requires a creative, strategic approach.

I finally understood that magic isn't something I do—it's something I engage with, something I interact with—when I became aware of what I perceive as a stream or current. I call it the *stream*. My great-aunt would always say, "Just do the thing (the spell), the spirits will come, and they know what to do." What she was expressing clicked for me when I realized that when we create—whether making art, cooking, sewing, or performing ritual—the best results come when we slip into the stream. I perceive this stream, this current, as a liminal space in motion that runs through all space and time, connecting us to our ancestors, ourselves, and our descendants. In this creative flow, their abilities, knowledge, experiences, and talents flow through us. To access them, we need to step into the stream, surrender to the current, and trust it to carry us forward. This stream of magic is the same one our ancestors accessed when they were alive, and now it exists in spirit form. This current is filled with everything—our ancestors' emotions, their hopes, dreams, fears, and joys; the saints, the gods, the demons. When we access it, we don't need to speak our intent aloud. By connecting with the stream, our spirits (ancestors) know exactly what we are requesting, and the request is granted—whether it comes as wisdom, a solution to a problem, or knowledge we need in that moment. This is how I understand divine providence—the flow of magic that's been available to us all along. It's not about forcing something to happen; it's about stepping into the current, surrendering to it, and trusting that it will carry us where we need to go.

Magical Practice Informs Profession/ Profession Informs Magical Practice

Magical practice informs profession, and profession informs magical practice. I live my magical practice, and folk magic is a living practice. Everything I do, I am always witching. I experience life and the world through the lens of my magical and spiritual practice. My magical skills are transferable to other areas of my life, and the skills I develop in my daily tasks also feed into my magic.

For example, when it comes to cooking and sewing, I approach every project with trust in the process. I apply the correct technique as I know it, but I am always open to the creative energy that flows through me. I observe how the ingredients or materials I am working with respond, and I work with them, not against them. Each project starts with an idea of what I want to create, but I remain open to the idea that it may take on a life of its own. I often say, "I never know exactly what I'm making until it's done."

I pay close attention to my thoughts, because sometimes a nudge will guide me in a different direction. I listen to the spirit of the project in the same way I listen to my plants and follow their guidance. Whatever your occupation, skills, or natural talents are, I am willing to bet they inform your magical practice, just as your magical practice informs them. You may not have realized this yet, but now you have. Living your folk magic practice means being engaged with it all the time—always witching. This is what it looks like when your folk magic is woven into every part of your life.

Chapter 4

Enchanted World
Animism in Folk Magic

The term *animism* derives from the Latin word *animus*, meaning spirit, soul, sentience. It names the perception and belief that all things, animate and nonanimate, living and nonliving, everything in nature and everything man-made is, in fact, *animated*—having agency and free will. Animism is not a religion but a worldview, and although it is not a religion in and of itself, it is the word used to describe what many believe is the most ancient understanding of human spirituality. As I understand and experience it, everything in my environment, seen or unseen, living or nonliving, has a spirit, and there is a supernatural power that animates the material universe.

In folk magic, animism isn't an abstract concept; it's the ground we stand on. It's the understanding that the world is alive with presence, filled with persons of all kinds: human and animal, tree and river, wind and fire, spirit and stone. As Dr. Graham Harvey explains in his book *Animism: Respecting the Living World*, animists recognize that life is always lived in relationship. He reminds us that animism isn't just about belief; it's about behaving well in a world of many beings and learning how to be a good person among them. In the context of folk magic, this means treating our tools, ingredients, ancestors, land, and spirits as relationships to be honored, not objects to be used.

Although animism works differently according to different cultures and people, this is how I approach it. I first came across the word *animism* in the context of anthropology. I recognized myself in it—though not completely at first. As I continued researching, gathering insights, and speaking with others who shared similar views, I came to a realization: I've been an animist for as long as I can remember. In truth, I believe we all begin that way—seeing the world as alive, connected, and full of presence.

Let me explain what I mean. Animism is at the heart of all the fairy tales my mother read to me when I was very young. Animism was depicted in all my favorite books and in all my favorite television characters. Through children's stories, movies, and television shows, children discover the world they live in and learn how to interact with and have empathy for other persons (human and nonhuman, animate and nonanimate, living and nonliving). Children's stories and movies and television, when done right, introduce children to abstract concepts of right and wrong in a secular framework of morality and ethics.

When I was a child, I perceived everything in nature as individual persons, and I interacted with them. Children naturally interact with animals, insects, plants, rocks, weather, the sun, and the moon. I am willing to guess that most likely you did too. All the stories and characters geared toward children are animistic. Seamlessly blending the natural and the supernatural cannot feel more natural to me, and it is such a fundamental piece in teaching children about the world. It begins with dolls, bedtime stories, and cartoons where the characters are other than humans and are all sentient or not sentient but persons nonetheless and very real to us. Animism is our first experience of spirituality. Does a child give their doll a name and personality, or does the toy reveal its name and personality to the child? I think about this a lot.

Our language reveals so much about our (humankind's) perception of and relationship to our world. We use adjectives that ascribe emotions to nature in sayings such as "the sea was angry that day." I want you to think back to your earliest memories. How did you perceive your environment? Did objects reveal their personalities to you? Did you have a favorite rock or some other object that felt like a dear friend and went with you everywhere? In accessing those memories, you can access that state of "knowing" that you had long ago. Accessing it and bringing it forth into your present will enrich your current practice.

I have experienced having that "knowing," losing it, and rediscovering it again firsthand. I recall feeling utterly alone in my teens, and my life was nothing but pointless hardship and emptiness. I did not believe the omniscient and omnipotent God of my Roman Catholic upbringing cared what we did or didn't do. Nor did I believe He spent His days granting rewards and meting out punishments. I couldn't believe a being so immense and powerful was micromanaging the banal lives of every single being on the planet. Shit didn't happen for a reason. Shit just happened, and a lot of it was shit. It was a liminal space where I didn't believe in fate (fatalism). I did not even believe in free will. Everything was random chance, and random chance was brutally unpredictable and ultimately senseless. Every defeat solidified and validated my hopelessness.

Then one fateful day during a physics lecture in college, I had a spiritual experience. The professor presented to the class how the entire universe is made up of two basic components: matter and energy. I was struck by the fact that most of the matter in the universe is invisible, and the source of most of the energy is not understood. What I heard was that matter and energy were indeed quantifiable. The source of the energy is not understood. I felt this in my bones, and this thought would proceed to haunt me for years. It is what sent me on my journey toward gaining meaning in my life and a profound sense of belonging in the universe and the desire to interact with all the persons who inhabit it and the supernatural power that organizes and animates us all. Only when I began to collect information from my relatives and neighbors on Italian folk practices did I learn that animism is not only at the root of ancient Italian folk beliefs, but according to conversations I had with my elders, they did not perceive a separation between their earth-and-land-spirit-based spirituality and their religion.

Over the years I have heard both praise and criticism when it comes to the blending of the sacred and the profane in Italian folk magic. The inclusion of the sacred (Catholicism) seems to be the contentious issue with people approaching this practice from a more Pagan perspective. On the other hand, devout Catholics raised practicing the folk ways that blend the sacred and the profane are just as put off by anyone pointing out that "the things they do" are not quite inside the lines of Catholicism. On further probing, I learned that what they really feared was angering "any" spirit (either known or unknown to them) that had power over their survival. For the longest time, I viewed Italian folk magic (or any cultural folk magic for that matter) as this simple bizarre love triangle consisting of cultural practices of benign magic, superstition and baneful magic, and their religion. Although this may be true on the surface, it is not the complete picture of what a living and breathing folk magic practice consists of. To be a folk magic practitioner means to have a fundamental belief that our world is animated (full of spirits) and to have the ability to interact with and coordinate these forces in a mutually beneficial way to effect change.

What I imagine is going on when I perform a spell or ritual is something like the Law of Conservation of Mass viewed from the perspective of animism. For those of you who may not know, I will give a very brief explanation. The Law of Conservation of Mass dates from Antoine Lavoisier's 1789 discovery that mass is neither created nor destroyed in chemical reactions. In other words, the mass of any one element at the beginning of a chemical reaction will equal the mass of that element at the end of the reaction, even if it has changed state. States of matter are solid, liquid, and gas.

What piqued my interest is that the formulation of this law was of critical importance in the forward movement from alchemy to the modern natural science of chemistry. I am not a scientist, and there is a possibility that I may not have gotten this description completely right. Neither am I proposing to give a scientific explanation as to what is going on during spell work. What I am proposing is that, for me, it is necessary to conceptualize what is happening even if it is only a metaphor. The metaphor allows me to consistently structure my spells and rituals in such a manner that I understand how it will attain the desired result. It does not have to be true because there is no way I can verify if this is truly how it works. It must *feel* true to me so I can believe in the process. Belief is what gives me sight, versus seeing is believing.

Here is an example using a simple candle spell. Candle wax houses its spirit. Its physical body is moldable, changing states between solid, liquid, and gas as fire is applied to it via a wick. The candle is prepared by carving words and symbols into it, and there may be words spoken to it. The spirit of the candle has been petitioned in addition to any other spirits one may have involved in this working. The candle is anointed with an oil (or not), and then it is lit. Since my metaphor is the Law of

Conservation of Mass, the mass of the candle is not destroyed. As the candle burns, the wax changes state to liquid and gas, at which point the spirit of the wax is released. The spirit of the wax is now free to embody or partially embody the intention that we burned the candle to manifest.

All magic comes at a cost. In this example, the candle is the sacrifice because we burned the candle in exchange for what we needed or wanted. This principle ties right in with the Italian folkloric practice of exchange when it comes to magic—exchanging one thing for another. For example, in ancient Abruzzese folk medicine, a live frog was bandaged to the forehead of a patient with a high fever. When the frog died from what they believed was absorbing the illness/fever, it was replaced with another until the illness/fever subsided. In essence, the lives of frogs were traded for the life of a human. The animist mentality of these people is clearly seen here when the lives of frogs are considered valuable currency to exchange for a human life.

Animism is the spiritual foundation of my folk witchery. I am firmly present in the material world while at the same time aware of and in communion with spirits who inhabit both the material and immaterial worlds. I have learned not to discount nor underestimate. In fact, I have learned to value more the love and support (and the power) of what I call more immediate spirits. These spirits inhabit my home and the land where I live. Other spirits consist of my ancestors and saints.

There is an interdependence between the folk witch and their spirits. They work together for mutually beneficial desired outcomes. These spirits may be human and nonhuman. It is perfectly natural for me to engage simultaneously with animal and plant spirits as well as ancestors and saints. They are as much a part of my family as is my living family. I do not compartmentalize my folk magic practice and my mundane life. It is all just how I live.

Enchanted Worldview

I have heard over and over again the phrase "an enchanted worldview" applied to people who practice a cultural folk magic tradition. Maybe I misunderstand or read too much into this expression, but it seems a bit infantilizing to me. I hear it as saying that folk magic practitioners all share a romanticized fairy-tale view of the world, the implication being that their worldview consists of a childlike naïveté, that the "low" magic they practice is pretend play. Again, I may be reading too much into it. I may have fixated on it a little too much, but I pulled on that thread, and at the end of it, I found a better way to describe our worldview. It is not our worldview (lens) that is enchanted; it is our view of the world (our ability to see) that the world is enchanted. Our magic lies in our ability to connect to and live in right relationship with the spirits who enchant the world.

Man-made structures are all made from elements derived from the natural world. It would stand to reason that the resulting structures would contain the spirits of their components or an entirely unique spirit of its own. If I had to name just one man-made object that I have had a long-standing relationship with, it is my car. I have had my current car now for over seventeen years. I take care of her, and she gets me where I need to go and keeps me safe. I have had many a close call commuting on winding mountain roads through inclement weather, and she has never let me down.

Similarly, electronic devices, appliances, and the like all have a spirit and their own personalities. I once observed my uncle talk to a machine that wasn't working, and then he would do something that appeared totally useless like applying a piece of tape to it, and suddenly, it was working again. When I asked him how he fixed something, because I wanted to learn how to fix things, he looked at me and replied, "Talk to it. Ask it what it needs and do it." Okay, so here is what I have learned over the last thirty years. If I ask my home, appliance, machine, or whatever that is not working what is wrong with it, it will tell me. Mostly in the form of a thought popping in my head and sometimes with an obvious sign. Nowadays, when something is not functioning, I ask it to help me help it. Sometimes the fix is obvious, other times not so much.

What I find shocking is how well electronic devices and appliances respond to the cure to dispel the evil eye. Years ago, right before a very important presentation, my old laptop wouldn't boot up. I knew she would soon need to be replaced, but I really needed her on that specific day. I completely powered her off, unplugged her, cleaned every inch externally, and performed the cure to dispel the evil eye. I told her to rest and that I would need her later that day and how important it was to me for her to show up. I bet you think I'm little crazy right now. That's fine. I'm perfectly okay with that. Otherwise, I wouldn't be sharing this story with you. After a little rest, fifteen minutes prior to the start of my presentation, I plugged her back in and pressed the power button. My laptop started without a hitch. It was like she hadn't been twitchy and flashing the blue screen the last three months. She performed remarkably well for my presentation, and she went on to perform nearly perfectly for another eighteen months afterward. This is just one example of my many experiences with fixing something by talking to it and performing the evil eye cure. I do this regularly at home and at work. The thing is, even after decades of using this fix regularly, when I do this and it works, or even better, when I suggest it to someone else and it works, that feeling of awe and wonder never gets old.

I believe that my primary relationship is with myself. When there is harmony between my mind, body, and spirit, accessing other spirits in my environment feels effortless. My environment can be external, internal, this plane or other planes of existence, etc. As an animist, I perceive myself as a member of a community of persons, both living and nonliving, human and nonhuman. The times in my life when I have suffered were when I had forgotten that although I am a solitary practitioner, I am not alone. We suffer when we forget that we belong to each other.

Years ago, I felt a strong need to simplify my life, and the first area of my life I needed to simplify was my magico-spiritual practice. Not that it was overly complicated; it was just the area of my life I felt needed more focus. Specifically, my spiritual beliefs. My spiritual beliefs are not static. They are formed, informed, and reformed by my spiritual (and mundane) experiences. Something I may have believed for decades may no longer fit following an experience or information that disproves my belief or prompts me to think or feel differently. Whenever this occurs, I use an exercise to check in with myself. On a sheet of paper—it has to be on paper with nice pens because I need the both the visual and tactile experience—I map out in words and symbols what my current spiritual life and beliefs look like. Once I have this information down on paper, I go on an exploration and ponder these practices and beliefs. I ask myself questions such as "Are they still true? Are they still relevant? Are they still meaningful? If not, what has changed? What needs to change?" This is a great way to gauge what we still value and what we may have outgrown. At first, the process feels weird and there is always some resistance, but I push through and as soon as I write down a few words, the rest begins to flow. I am always amazed at how this simple exercise can bring clarity and have such a profound impact, resulting in a recalibration of sorts. I recommend this simple but powerful exercise whenever anyone wishes to regain focus and understanding with respect to their spirituality. In fact, whether you are just setting out on your journey to build your own folk magic practice, or you have been practicing for a while, I recommend you stop right here and do this exercise.

Here is a list of introspective prompts for your folk magic practice and spiritual beliefs:

What are the core spiritual beliefs that resonate deeply within me and feel undeniably true?

How do these beliefs manifest and express themselves in my daily life?

What elements of my environment help me feel more spiritually connected?

What practices or actions do I engage in that bring me closer to my spiritual self?

What is the one thing I hold above all else in life, and why is it so important to me?

How do I perceive and define folk magic in my life and practice?

What motivates me to practice folk magic, and why do I feel compelled to continue this path?

What influences shape my magical practice—be it my cultural background, ancestral connections, nature, or spirits?

What are my personal ethics and boundaries when it comes to practicing magic? What feels right to me, and what do I avoid?

Chapter 5

Building Sacred Bonds
Cultivating Relationships with Spirits

Spirit Allies and Enemies, Friends and Foes

Over the course of many years, and a lot of trial and error, I have learned a few things about developing and maintaining relationships with spirits. One of my biggest takeaways so far when it comes to spirits that used to be human is how similar these relationships are to relationships with the living. I am most familiar with ancestors and saints. Let's start with ancestors.

While this is certainly not unique to my culture, we believe that our immediate ancestors—primarily our parents, grandparents, followed by aunts, uncles, and cousins we may have been close with, as well as chosen family—continue to be present and interested in our lives. They continue to participate in our lives, providing guidance and protection. It is a given, per our beliefs, that these ancestors are in our spirit court. I have come to appreciate that it is their jobs to have our backs, whether we want to continue maintaining our relationship with them or not.

Let me explain. We can live entirely full lives without any interest or interactions with the spirits. What I am referring to is the matter of which ancestors we wish to stay or get in touch with. The thing with ancestors that we knew in life is that relationships can be very complicated and, in some cases, deeply disappointing and downright disorienting. I have found that this is mostly due to our own expectations and lack of understanding and, in some cases, common sense. To put it simply, families are complex organisms. If the ancestors that we knew in life did not have our best interests at heart when they were living, perhaps they shouldn't be the first ones we call on the (figuratively speaking) spirit phone when we need help. Nor are we obligated to honor or maintain relationships with ancestors who may have acted heinously when they were alive. The act of dying did not magically turn them into angels or saints. I have learned that, just as in life some people are not for us, some dead are not for us. In my experience, it is possible to gain a better understanding of and approach forgiveness toward an ancestor after they've died. Our relationship, once truly stripped of all the noise, drama, and baggage of the mundane world, can take on a direct heart-to-heart, soul-to-soul quality that leaves space for the truth and, with time, can be conducive to healing both parties—the living and the dead. I have had one such relationship for the last twenty years. This relationship has taught me a lot about grief and forgiveness. In the case of this relationship, I learned that when someone dies, we grieve the love we never received from them, the love we never got to give and will never get to give, and the relationship we never had.

There is a cultural custom I once thought was unique to my family: When someone is nearing the end of their life, a loved one will ask them to promise to visit from the afterlife. As a palliative care nurse, I have since witnessed this same request across many cultures and religious beliefs around the world.

When my father was dying and still conscious, I visited him at the hospital. After I sat by his bedside for what felt like hours while he rested, he woke up, surprised to see me still there. He let out a big sigh and said, "I'm dying, Mary-Grace."

I simply replied, "I know." Then I asked him to promise me something. I asked, "When you're gone, will you come back and visit me? And tell me whatever you can about where you are?"

He perked up immediately and said, "Of course, I will! You think if I can do that I won't?"

I answered, "I know you. It's the one thing I'm asking of you. Please, do it."

This experience brought to light a truth: Building relationships with the spirits of people we knew in life can be just as complicated as the relationships we had when they were alive. Expectations can cloud these connections. So, if you feel called to it, by all means, reach out to them. But, just as with the living, it's important to approach this situation with open eyes. My advice is to be cautiously optimistic and set healthy boundaries, keeping your expectations in check. And just in case you're wondering, three months after my father passed, he did indeed keep his promise.

The next spirits are ancestors in our bloodline whom we have never met, or maybe we were far too young to remember them when we did meet. This type also includes ancestors who lived and died long before we were born. These spirits are, in my opinion, easier to approach because we don't have a history with them. We may have a photo. We may know some things about them. We may have neither. In my personal experience, I have found it easy to connect to spirits of my maternal ancestors, even though (or perhaps because) I know very little about them. I have always found that very interesting.

I also want to share that when I speak of ancestors, I don't mean merely those in the "old country" for those of us who were not born and raised in the land of our ancestors. There are also our ancestors in the diaspora. Ancestors of our family, community, and chosen families. Ancestors of shared experiences—that is, immigration, occupation, trade, art, interests, hobbies, spirituality, magic, religion. Some ancestors are related by blood, others by love.

Ancestors and Culture

Our ancestors' magic and spirituality were not viewed as separate from their mundane lives. Their skills, knowledge, experience, beliefs, and superstitions were crucial to the survival of their descendants and the continuation of their culture. Oral tradition was (and still is) transmitted via fantastic and mystical stories and allegories, and for the most part, all unverifiable personal experience and gnosis. The proof was always in the successful outcome of the spell or ritual and predictions coming true. We need to be comfortable with this if we wish to live our lives magically.

To be in a relationship with our ancestors, we need to meet them on their terms. We need to have a grasp of their context and cultural understanding because the world was a very different place when they were alive. The more we understand and embrace this, the more we will be able to engage, connect, and participate in clear communication with them. Expecting these spirits to behave in a manner consistent with our modern-day sensibilities and sociocultural ideologies is not helpful and may only create unnecessary barriers in communication. Such expectations only create confusion for all involved.

When seeking their assistance, what I have found works best is to connect with them on the level of concerns related to survival. Needs related to our survival are timeless. Love is eternal. Our ancestors may have had political views contrary to ours when they were alive, but they 100 percent can relate to our needs for survival. My Italian grandmother, who was born in 1898 and lived her entire life in a tiny town in the mountains of central Italy, can certainly relate to my need to find a job because it means survival. It does not benefit me to need my grandmother's approval of my personal life choices that she may not have agreed with in life. I just need her love and support. At the same time, I cannot assume that my grandmother would not understand my personal life choices either. The arrogance of youth made me think that no one older than me had any idea what I was going through. With age and experience, I gained the understanding that not only did they have an idea, but they also went through it too and in some cases even worse than I did. It benefits me to maintain an open mind that she, understanding my circumstances, will come to my aid because she "gets" it, and love transcends all that. The biological fact remains that they are literally part of us. We literally carry parts of them within us, as we are made up partially of their DNA. It doesn't matter if we never knew our ancestors; we are linked to them through the cells in our bodies. Your ancestors are in your spirit court whether you know who they are or not. But don't discount your ancestors who are not linked to you through blood but through love. You are not alone.

Since our genetic makeup contains that of our ancestors, I have always pondered past lives' memories versus our ancestors' memories, so-called genetic memories. What is mine? What is theirs? What is the collective?

Saints: To clarify, when I refer to saints, I am referring to the wide variety of saints, sages, mystics, prophets, folk saints, shamans, and so on. All cultures have holy ancestors who were religiously and culturally significant and influential when they were alive and continued to have this influence from the spirit world. I view saints as ancestors. My approach in connecting with and developing a new relationship with saints consists of finding out what I can about their lives. They used to be human, so learning about their lives allows me to form a connection with them as people. It allows me to imagine them living mundane lives, which makes them so much more relatable for me. We have access to historical accounts about the lives of our holy ancestors through books. Nowadays a quick Internet search can provide just as much if not more information on the life of our holy ancestor and also the geography of where they were and the history of their culture.

The first saints I connected with were the patron saints of my ancestors. They were introduced to me at a very young age as "our" saints. Patron saints of the villages in Italy where my family came from. Patron saints of their occupations and the saints they petitioned regularly who always interceded. In time, I forged my own relationships with saints and spirits who made themselves known to me or I reached out to out of necessity. It is my feeling that since saints were once human, they are accessible to everyone regardless of religion. I have lost count of how many times I have heard someone who is not Catholic praise a saint who helped them.

My experience has been that saints, unlike the living people in our lives, do not grow tired of our requests for their help and, in fact, are quite welcoming and supportive. There is no such thing as asking for help too often, but there are some caveats. Bombarding our patron saint with numerous different requests confuses us more than it may confuse them and may result in a bit of a mess. It is better to focus on the most urgent and important matter so that we can best hear or perceive their guidance.

When you ask for help, trust that help is already granted. Our patron saint is not rigidly assigned a specific niche. If your patron saint is documented to be the patron saint of cobblers, for example, and you have a solid relationship with them, they are certainly qualified to help with other matters. When I need help, I always turn to my patron saint, the one I am closest to, even if it is not their "specialty," and get excellent results. On the other hand, I wouldn't recommend asking for help with things we can certainly do ourselves without their assistance. Learned helplessness is a hindrance that can keep us stuck waiting for them to solve all our problems. Do the work, and your spirits will come to your aid.

Nonhuman spirits: The nonhuman spirits in my life are the ones I have the most daily contact with. I am not exactly sure why, but I think the reason might have something to do with me being introverted. Examples of nonhuman spirits are elemental spirits of air, fire, water, and earth. These also include forces of nature and weather, fae, plus animal and plant spirits. I view them collectively as spirits of the land (that also may include ancient spirits of former humans).

Ancestral spirits hold a significant place in folk traditions across cultures, often serving as guides, protectors, and sources of wisdom for the living. Many believe that the spirits of deceased family members continue to influence the world, offering blessings or requiring rituals to ensure harmony. Guardian ancestors are thought to watch over their descendants, protecting them from harm and guiding their choices. Mediator ancestors act as intermediaries between the living and other spiritual beings, helping convey prayers or warnings. Ancestor spirits provide guidance through dreams, divination, or trance states. Offerings often involve rituals consisting of food, drink, or incense to honor and, depending on the culture, appease ancestral spirits. Ancestor spirits can be bringers of fortune or misfortune. Honored ancestors are believed to bring good luck, while neglected spirits may cause illness or misfortune as a sign of displeasure.

Each culture has its own unique relationship to ancestral spirits, and every practitioner will have their own unique relationship to their ancestral spirits.

Here are some examples from different cultures:

- In Chinese ancestral veneration, families offer incense and food, and burn paper money to honor ancestors, especially during festivals like Qingming.
- In some Nigerian and many other African traditions, ancestral spirits are highly respected, with libations and rituals performed to seek their guidance. Offerings of food, water, and other goods are presented to ancestors at designated shrines or burial sites to seek their guidance, protection, and blessings.
- Mexican Día de los Muertos (Day of the Dead) is the day when families create altars (*ofrendas*) with offerings to welcome the spirits of their ancestors.
- In Slavic cultures, rituals such as Dziady (Forefathers' Eve) are observed by Belarusians, Poles, Ukrainians, and Lithuanians. This communion of the living and the dead involves honoring ancestors with offerings of food and candlelit prayers.

There are numerous ways to connect with ancestral spirits. The most commonly practiced tradition is setting up an ancestral altar with photos, candles, and offerings. Others are honoring family traditions and storytelling to keep ancestral wisdom alive as well as celebrating cultural festivals dedicated to honoring our ancestors.

Then there is the practice of ancestral meditation or dreamwork to receive messages. What I share is the practice I developed for myself. Mine is not the only way to do something. I share to inspire you to cook up your own practice.

Connecting and Maintaining Relationships

The Ones You Know

Let's begin with ancestors that we knew in life. They include blood relatives, nonrelatives, and friends. To connect with an ancestor I knew in life, the first thing I do is think about them. That is usually enough to feel their presence. I can feel their presence through a shift in energy, and it feels like them, picturing them in my mind, or physical sensations like that of a hand just barely touching my arm or simply feeling my heart fill with love. If I just want to connect to say hello and let them know I am thinking about them, this is all I do. When I miss them, I invite them for a cup of tea and just sit with them for a little while. It never gets old how I feel their energy when they arrive, and I can feel when they go. Some visits are shorter than I would like them to be. Experience has taught me that this is not at all up to me. No matter how hard I concentrate, I can't make them stay longer. They come when I call, and they leave of their own accord, but they are always within reach.

Another way I connect with them is when I am engaged in an activity we used to do together. I begin by thinking about how we used to do the activity together and ask them to join me. This is a wonderful way to connect with your ancestors when you need to confide in someone you trust or can use their support and advice. Just talk to them. We can connect with our ancestors by talking to their photo or while holding or wearing an object that used to belong to them. At first, you may feel ridiculous or as though you are making it all up. Keep doing it; keep practicing. Trust this process. This is the most direct and effective way to connect to them.

Mundane tasks like physical labor and household chores are the liminal spaces where we commune with our ancestors. They provide cover (we're busy doing something) and mental space to interact with our ancestors to ask for support and advice related to concerns in our lives. Alternatively, we may just want to visit with loved ones. Sometimes the living are reaching out; other times the dead are dropping in.

Another thing we can do when we want to connect with our dearly departed is to light a candle. I was taught from a very young age that when we light a candle, the flame is visible to the spirit world. In essence, we are contacting the spirit world in the hope that our ancestors see the light and respond. When electric lights dim on their own or when you see flashes of light in your peripheral vision, ask if your ancestors are contacting you. When you do this, ask them to repeat the sign.

Dreams are the most common way my elders reported receiving messages from the dead. One relative wrote entire letters to them and then tossed the letters in the fire. Another one placed bits of paper with short messages in a tin box that once held chocolates and was kept just for this purpose. The letters and messages were sent, and these relatives went on with their lives. They knew not to wait impatiently for the dead to answer them. The dead always answered them through dreams, in their own time. The dead had other ways to reply as well. It was also common for answers to come via a quick exchange with a random stranger. For example, a random stranger might stop them in public and say something that sounded totally cryptic until they got home and remembered the message they had sent.

One of my aunts always dreamt of the dead. All the dead relatives (and her neighbors) visited her on a nightly basis. She often relayed messages that were independently and objectively verifiable. However, and this is a big however, my aunt was also very religious, and so were many of her neighbors. I suspect that dreams of the dead are common because dreams are involuntary and thus not witchcraft. This aunt saying she dreamt of her neighbor telling her to tell his widow that the important documents she needed were under a floorboard was much more likely to be well received (and without suspicion) than "Your husband's spirit appeared to me in my parlor, and he asked me to tell you he hid the deed to the house under the floorboard under his side of the bed."

My other aunt lamented (with a lot of jealousy) that no one visited her in her dreams. The dead would "just appear," and because they would just appear to her, when she shared her experiences, her reported experiences were viewed as less credible and discounted. Well-meaning friends and family would express concern that she was imagining things, and they would warn her to be careful that most likely malefic spirits were tempting her.

I bring up this story because when I was less experienced, these types of rigid beliefs about what was "real" spirit communication and what was not really hindered me. Trust me when I tell you that you will have your own unique experiences. They may or may not be exactly like someone else's. You do not need to prove or even tell anyone anything about your intimate and sacred relationships with your spirits. Maintaining relationships with the spirits of the dead requires effort and an open mind on our part. The effort is worthwhile though. This is how the dead participate in our mundane lives. Another way of keeping in touch with our ancestors and keeping their memories alive is by sharing their stories at every occasion when family is gathered.

The Ones You Don't Know

What if you want to connect with ancestors you don't know? These ancestors can be family members who lived long before you were born or ancestors who were alive in your lifetime but you never met. For our purpose here, this includes any ancestors you have never met regardless of when they lived. I have attempted this type of contact a few times with mixed results. Each time my reason for attempting to contact an ancestor I don't know has been to try to piece together family history in the hopes of gaining a better understanding of who I am. I feel that this is common among people who are searching to know more about where they came from. My mixed results had much to do with my somewhat unrealistic expectations. I thought that connecting with unknown ancestors would give me answers. Instead, it left me with way more questions.

Allow me to walk you through my best experience. This part is important because it illustrates how we need to trust our own feelings in this type of work. I did not know this ancestor in life. They died a long time before I was born. I had a name and an old photo that a family member confirmed was in fact them. I began by asking other family members about this ancestor. As much as anyone knew. None of my family members knew this ancestor either. They only knew of them. So, I had a name, a photo, and some very vague information about where they were from and when they died. The photo was small, so I carried it around in my wallet. Once a day I would take some time, ten or fifteen minutes, to just think about them. I probably should mention that all this stuff that I do—and did—is all self-taught. There was no Internet, and even if there was a book on connecting with ancestors at that time, I did not know about it.

Every day, whenever I remembered to, I would take ten to fifteen minutes to think of this family member. I repeated this routine for months. To my dismay, they did not visit me in a dream. What I did experience was even weirder. While I was watching a TV show, out of nowhere, something in the plot matched up with what I knew about my ancestor. Some kind of parallel story. In this episode, it was revealed that the main character never knew their father, and the little they did know about him matched almost exactly the little I knew about the ancestor whom I was trying to connect with. Now the show had my attention. I watched the episode with goosebumps all over my body and my heart racing. In the show, the character finally learned details about their father, where he was from (which matched my ancestor), his occupation (because it was very specific and unusual, I made note of it because it matched the little I knew of my ancestor), and how he met his demise. Less than a month later, I attended a relative's funeral. There I was introduced to an elderly woman because she hailed from the same town as my relatives. She looked at my face and said I must be related to ___, the same ancestor I had been trying to contact. I quickly asked her how she knew them and if she could tell me anything about them. The information she gave me was consistent with what I already knew, and here's the kicker: The additional information about my ancestor was exactly, and I mean *exactly*, the same as the character's father in the TV show I had watched. I considered that to be confirmation of connection with my ancestor. This experience felt so much bigger and more meaningful than it looks on paper. I connected to my ancestor, and I felt that connection in every fiber of my being. I have made other attempts to connect with ancestors I don't know over the years, but none of those experiences were like this one.

In daily practice, my ancestors and spirits are consultants, confidants, and family members. I honor them, but I do not worship them so that I do not place myself in a mental state of helplessness. The danger of becoming so reliant and viewing yourself as helpless without them is very real and can result in your giving up agency. To connect with them, I turn inward instead of outward and on display. I don't need to phone them daily on the spirit phone to say, "I'm thinking of you." They let me know when they are around, and I acknowledge and thank them. I know what I want. I know what I need. I honor their memory by sharing their stories the same way my parents shared the stories of their grandparents and great-grandparents. The storytelling is composed of all the vicissitudes of life—the good, the bad, the happy (joys), the sad (sorrows), fortune and misfortune, tragedy, the beauty and ugliness of their lives and experiences. I can't help but be aware that I too will one day be an ancestor. What am I leaving behind? What am I passing down?

Nonhuman Spirits

I refer to the countless spirits that were, in our understanding, never previously human as nonhuman spirits (animal spirits, plant spirits, elemental spirits, land spirits, spirits of place, spirits from other worlds, and so on). This is a very loose description of these spirits because I honestly don't feel qualified to classify them at all. All I am hoping to accomplish is to make the distinction between the spirits that I perceive as having experience and understanding of the human condition and those that do not. I don't mean it in the sense that they are all lumped together in one category. I also use this descriptor to indicate that how I connect and maintain my relationship with these spirits is much different from how I connect and maintain a relationship with human spirits. To be honest, I am not quite sure who or what they are. I accept them as is, and it seems they are fine with that acceptance.

Communicating with nonhuman spirits begins with perceiving their presence. It requires paying close attention with all our senses to learn the subtle and not-so-subtle differences in their energies. Connecting with these spirits requires a different set of communication skills (images, thoughts, other cues). I find it similar to communicating with living plants and animals or like meeting someone from a different country whose language you do not understand. You learn to communicate nonverbally through gestures and common words in both your languages until you gradually learn each other's language enough to meet each other halfway.

These are the spirits I work with most closely in my magical practice. These are the spirits I interact with daily. These are the spirits that connect me to my environment. They are my constant companions, but they don't exist to serve me, nor do I serve them. The relationship is very much like good neighbors. We coexist interdependently. I treat them with respect, and in turn, they are very keen to help and, to my surprise, are fiercely protective of me and everyone I love.

Nonhuman spirits can be fiercely loyal and protective of us. They may seek vengeance for the slightest injustices done to you of their own volition and without your request or accord. First, a little warning: Exercise extreme caution when asking these spirits for their help. Make sure you use very clear language that is absent of emotion. If you say something in a heightened emotional state that you really didn't mean, it may not be possible to explain to these spirits "I really didn't mean it that way"—especially because of the emotional energy attached to what you said. Always keep in mind that these spirits don't get nuance. Say only what you mean or say nothing at all. Aside from that little caveat, these spirits are my favorites.

What I find the most fascinating with nonhuman spirits is that the more you acknowledge and appreciate them, the more they want to help. My relationship with these helper spirits has taught me so much about interdependence and reciprocity. My helpers are my ground troops, and they look out for me because I, in turn, take care of them. Our relationships are based in mutual respect. Because they are incorporeal, spirits have certain advantages. Because humans are corporeal, we have certain advantages. Think of the possibilities when we work together and combine our advantages.

The most essential tool in my magical tool kit is not a physical tool but a skill. Spirit communication is a skill that anyone can learn. Like any skill, it requires dedication to learning and practice. What I think of when I say "communicating with spirit" is the ability to feel their presence, dialogue, and collaborate with them.

A Word on Working with Spirits

The phrase "working with spirits" is used a lot by all types of magic and witchcraft practitioners, and I am not sure what it means to other people; therefore, I want to share with you what it means to me. When I work with spirits, literal work is involved. I am doing the work of carrying out tasks in the physical world for myself and on behalf of my spirits. This is what I mean when I say I work with spirits. When I help someone by holding space for them while they work on finding their way back after losing their sense of self, I am working with Saint Anthony of Padua. When I am taking care of my pets and ensuring there is plenty of fresh water for the wildlife and the plants in my backyard, I am working with the spirits of the land.

What does taking care of my spirits look like? If I were to describe the vast majority of what I do to maintain my relationships and take care of my spirits, it would probably be a combination of stewardship and hospitality. These spirits are all welcome here, and I make sure they know it. How do I show them this is a place where they're welcome and honored? I take care of my living spaces, and in turn, this creates a welcoming environment for the spirits who occupy my living spaces. I carry out acts of service. My acts of service are offerings to my spirits. Acts of service can be caring for my elderly German Shepherd, leaving my backyard to grow wild for pollinators and visiting woodland creatures, or making sure the bird bath has clean, fresh water daily. I take care of my houseplants, and their spirits watch over us. I include my ancestors by telling their stories and describing what I think their reaction would be to an event if they were present.

With practice, we develop our own code to contact spirits and our own ways to maintain our relationships with them. Some spirits are daily-contact type friends; others are contacted as needed. We must be comfortable with feeling a connection without knowing for sure, without validation from an external party. But there will be signs, irrefutable signs that, although they cannot be proven, you feel in your bones, in your blood, to be true.

Animals in Folk Practice

Interactions with living animals, pets, wild animals, and bugs were my gateway to animal spirits and are still the largest component of my spiritual practice. I was very little when I began talking to animals. Cartoons on TV taught me animals are just like people, so why wouldn't I believe it? All the grown-ups I knew talked to animals, and I saw how the animals responded. My mom spoke to our dog the same way she spoke to me or anyone else. I remember being in my playpen and my mom telling our German Shorthaired Pointer Dora to watch me and call her if I was trying to climb out. I also remember the sting of betrayal when Dora finked on me. We said good morning to the squirrels in our backyard and the bugs in our garden.

I am willing to bet that this is a very common thing that no one talks about. Animals and bugs are not cartoon characters, and although our communication with them may be verbal, they communicate back nonverbally. When I pay attention to animal behaviors, both domestic and wild, there is always a message. I perceive animal spirits as both the incorporeal spirits of animals and the essence or life force of living animals. When my animal guardian spirits want to communicate with me, their live counterparts will interact with me, and there is no mistaking this communication for anything other than messages from spirit. It is all animal spirit to me, and I do not differentiate between the living and nonliving.

Years ago, I had an experience that shaped my understanding. It was not uncommon for me to see quite a variety of wildlife on the main highway on my commute to work. To one side of this highway is the lake; on the other side, the mountains. Every time that I spotted roadkill, I sent a blessing to the spirit of the animal. Every time animals crossed in front of my car or flew over me, I acknowledged them and greeted them. I drove on this same highway daily for years and knew every inch of it. One morning, a sign that I saw every day and never gave any attention to really caught my eye. As I drove past it, on this morning, the image of that same sign flashed big and right in front of me like it was in my car! It read: "Watch for Wildlife." Okay, noted. I slowed down a bit and did what the sign commanded. When I arrived at my last turn down the street where I worked, it happened. I drove a bit slower and was paying close attention when I heard and saw the neighborhood crows I greeted every day all come down from a tree and land, covering the entire road in front of my car. I counted at least two dozen of them. The crows right in front of my car lay on the ground with their chests pressed down onto the pavement. I got out of my car to check if they were hurt. They didn't move. Even more strange was that no other cars or people were on that very busy road during the morning rush hour. The street was eerily deserted and silent. Even these usually very chatty crows were silent. The silence was deafening, and it felt like time stood still. Then, like someone flipped a switch, the crows got up and walked to the other side of the street, and some flew back up in the trees. I got back in my car and went to work. I made a quick voice recording on my phone of this experience and carried on with my day. I was a little freaked out because I, being an anxious person, immediately judged this to be a bad omen. It was not. Less than two months later, I would come to understand that this encounter was a message from my spirits that I had their fierce protection during what would be a very precarious time in my life. When we develop and maintain a relationship with animal spirits, we begin to be a steward of the animals in our care and the wildlife in our environments.

Animal Omens

Animal omens are signs or messages believed to be conveyed through the appearance or behavior of animals. Many cultures interpret these occurrences as predictions of future events, whether good or bad. The meaning of an animal omen varies based on the species, context, and cultural beliefs. For example, a black cat crossing one's path is often seen as a bad omen in Western traditions (although my personal experience has shown the opposite to be true), while an owl's call may signal wisdom or death. Some people view these signs as messages from spirits, ancestors, or deities, and thus they hold a lot of significance in folk spiritual practices.

The practice of reading animal omens is not confined to rural areas; these omens can be observed in urban settings as well. Birds flying into windows, stray animals behaving unusually, or insects appearing in unexpected places are often interpreted as signs, even in cities. Urban dwellers may associate these encounters with personal or cultural beliefs, just as those in rural areas do. The meaning of an omen depends on the observer's perspective and traditional interpretations.

Interpreting animal omens in folk practice requires understanding and combining your cultural beliefs, the animal's characteristics, and the context of the encounter. Here are some key steps to get you started:

Observe the animal and their behavior: Take note of the species, its actions, and any unusual behavior. A lone crow cawing may signify that you will receive news regarding a family member, while a deer appearing suddenly could mean that you need to maintain your boundaries.

Consider your cultural and regional beliefs: Different cultures assign different meanings to animals. For example, in some traditions, owls symbolize wisdom, whereas in others, they are omens of death.

Pay attention to timing and context: The time and place of the encounter can influence its meaning. If you are going through a major life transition, seeing an animal may indicate guidance or a warning.

Look for patterns and take note of repetition: If the same animal appears to you repeatedly, folk belief suggests the message is of greater importance and urgency. A recurring visit from a specific bird, for instance, could be seen as a message from a specific spirit or ancestor.

Reflect on your own personal and symbolic meanings: Your own experiences and feelings about an animal matter. If you spot a fox and the book you are referencing states it represents cunning but it reminds you of a cherished childhood memory, I have found the personal meaning is always the correct meaning for me. Trust your intuition and inner knowing. Omens are meant for the individual who sees them, so your gut feeling about an animal encounter holds the most significance.

Animal Spirit Guides

In many folk traditions, animal spirit guides (also known as totem animals or power animals, depending on the tradition) are believed to be spiritual beings that offer guidance, protection, and wisdom. These spirits often take the form of animals and are thought to connect with individuals based on their personality, life challenges, or spiritual path. Animal spirit guides act as messengers by bringing signs or warnings about future events. As protectors, they offer spiritual or physical protection in difficult times. They can serve as teachers providing lessons about strength, patience, or adaptability. They can assist in emotional or spiritual healing.

In many Indigenous cultures across North America—including Native American and Canadian First Nations traditions—it's understood that each person may have one or more animal spirit guides. These spirit allies offer teachings, protection, and strength, and are often revealed through dreams, vision quests, or other spiritual experiences. Clan animals and personal totems carry deep meaning, rooted in ancestral relationships with the land and spirit world.

In Celtic mythology, animals like the stag, raven, and wolf were seen as messengers from the Otherworld, guiding warriors, druids, and seekers.

Shamans worldwide, including (but not limited to) Siberian, African, and South American cultures, work with animal spirits during rituals and journeys to access wisdom or healing energy.

In Chinese and Japanese folklore, animals such as dragons, foxes (*kitsune*), and cranes are seen as spiritual beings that influence fate, wisdom, and transformation.

In Nordic and Germanic beliefs, animals like wolves (Odin's wolves, Geri and Freki) and ravens (Huginn and Muninn) were considered messengers between the physical and spiritual worlds.

We can connect with our animal spirit guides through meditation, dreams, or personal encounters with animals in nature.

Plant Spirits

I have a tight and mighty group of plant spirit allies. My relationships with them have been forged over decades of always working with the same ones. This was not intentional on my part. My fantasy self is one who spends all her time in a lush garden planting and caring for a wide variety of plants. My real self has a small variety of garden and houseplant spirit allies that protect my home and alert me when I need to beef up my defenses. I have plants that grow outside my home that protect my home and provide shelter and nourishment to the wildlife. Finally, I have a group of plant allies I use in my magic, medicine, and cooking.

Roles of Plant Spirits in Folk Magic

Many cultures believe that plants have spirits that provide healing. Folk witches who are also herbalists often work with these spirits to enhance the medicinal effects of herbs.

Some plants are used in folk magic to ward off evil or negative energies, such as garlic against evil spirits in European folklore or sage used for cleansing in North American Indigenous traditions.

Plants can be seen as messengers of omens or divine signs. For example, the sudden blooming of a certain flower might be considered a message from ancestors or spirits.

Some traditions use plant spirits in shamanic journeys, such as ayahuasca in Amazonian cultures or peyote in North American Indigenous spiritual practices.

Trees such as the oak, yew, and willow have deep spiritual meaning in many traditions, symbolizing wisdom, protection, and connection to the divine.

Examples from Different Cultures

- The Celts believed trees, especially oak and ash, had spirits and were portals to other realms.
- In Japanese Shinto tradition, trees and sacred groves are home to *kami* (spiritual beings), and some are marked with *shimenawa* (sacred ropes).
- In Italian and a variety of Slavic folk traditions, plants such as wormwood were used in rituals to protect against spirits or curses.
- In African and Caribbean traditions, baobab trees are seen as ancestral homes and sources of wisdom.
- In Chinese folk tradition, the peach tree is believed to have protective qualities against evil spirits.

Practices for developing relationships and working with plant spirits are very much like the practices we use to connect with other spirits. Meditation, burning or brewing herbs for spiritual insight and as offerings to other spirits, leaving offerings at sacred trees, and dream interpretation are related to plant encounters.

Chapter 6

Dreams, Trance, Spirit Flight, and Time Travel in Folk Magic

Often seen as messages from the spirit world, omens of the future, or reflections of a person's spiritual state, dreams have been deeply significant in folk traditions across cultures. There exist many unique beliefs and practices surrounding dreams, including interpretation methods, protective rituals, and prophetic meanings in all cultures. Some dreams are believed to be prophetic and foretell the future, revealing warnings, blessings, or important life events. Ancestors, deities, or other spiritual beings may send guidance or requests through dreams. Dreams also can be seen as a journey of the soul, where a person travels to other realms while sleeping. Many dream elements, such as animals, objects, or natural events, hold symbolic meanings based on cultural traditions. Some dreams provide insight into a person's health, emotional state, or spiritual progress. Nightmares and unsettling dreams may be interpreted as signs of curses, spiritual unrest, or unresolved issues.

The ancient Egyptians believed dreams were divine messages, and priests acted as dream interpreters and turned to the Dream Book to decipher the symbols within a dream. The Egyptian Dream Book is an ancient text that reveals the Egyptians' belief in dreams as divine messages. The text lists various dream symbols and their interpretations, offering insight into the guidance and omens that dreams could provide. For the ancient Egyptians, dreams weren't just fleeting images; they were considered sacred communications from the gods, shaping the way individuals navigated both their spiritual and earthly journeys.

Many North American Indigenous tribes believe dreams are sacred visions, often guiding shamans and warriors in their spiritual path. Dreamcatchers are believed to catch and filter out bad dreams. Originating with the Ojibwe people, these handcrafted objects are made with a circular frame and a woven web, often decorated with feathers and beads. The idea is that the dreamcatcher traps negative dreams and spirits in its web, keeping them away from the sleeper, while letting the good dreams pass through the center or slide down the feathers.

The ancient Greeks believed dreams were sent by the gods, with figures like Morpheus overseeing the dream world. Ancient Romans often recorded dreams to interpret them for omens.

Chinese folk beliefs surrounding dreams are that they are linked to energy (*qi*) and could reveal hidden truths or predict the future. Some believe the soul could leave the body during sleep.

In Islamic and Middle Eastern folk traditions, dreams are highly valued, with certain dreams considered direct messages from the divine. Islamic texts mention different categories of dreams, including true visions and misleading dreams.

In European folk customs, many believe dreams could reveal signs of witchcraft, curses, or impending events and are taken as serious warnings.

Despite regional differences, many cultures see dreams as powerful spiritual experiences that can provide warnings, guidance, or insight into the future. Whether through herbs, prayers, or symbolic actions, these rituals highlight the deep connection between dreams and the unseen world.

The Italian immigrants of my family and community shared a solid oral tradition regarding the appearance of the sacred in dreams and visions. The sacred appeared in their dreams in all forms from a saint to a beloved dead to an animal, a tree, or a body of water that had important significance to them. Dreams were their favorite topic of conversation, especially at the breakfast table, and their primary spiritual expression.

In my decades of personal practice, conversations with family members, and comparisons of my experiences to their experiences and what was passed down to them, I would come to understand that the term *dream* is what my ancestors used to describe what they dreamt when they were asleep, as well as what they "dreamt" when they were awake (visions, trance). They "dreamt" when their spirit traveled away from their bodies and met up with others (spirit flight). They visited the past and the future in their "dreams" (time travel). Dreams signified anything from aspirations to spirit flight.

I can't talk about dreams without talking about two main Italian superstitions regarding sleep. First, there is an Italian superstition that turns out is not just Italian: One should never sleep with their feet by the doorway into the room.

Historically, many cultures have had concerns about safety while sleeping. In times past, when personal safety was more precarious, the position of the body during sleep could influence the degree of protection perceived. Keeping the head a safe distance away from the entrance may be considered a safer option because it allows one to see who enters the room and react quickly in case of danger. However, the superstition is tied more to a sense of respect for the deceased. In some funeral traditions, it is very important to position the deceased with their feet facing out of the room to allow them to "exit" the earthly plane and "walk" over to the afterlife. Sleeping in such a position could be seen as a kind of imitation of this ritual, which could be considered disrespectful to the deceased or bring misfortune. The consensus is that, ideally, the head of the bed should be positioned against a solid, stable wall, preferably one that is as far away from the door as possible. This position provides a sense of stability and security while sleeping. The bed should be oriented so that you can see the door without being directly in line with it.

I have not yet found any definitive scientific explanation as to why you should not sleep with your feet toward the door, but only as a practice that has cultural roots and superstitions in many parts of the world. For this reason, anyone who wants to sleep with their feet facing the door is free to do so; the only risk is going against an ancient belief or tradition, which may lead others to judge you.

Second, there is also a superstition that says to avoid sleeping in front of mirrors. In many cultures the mirror is considered an open window to the afterlife; therefore, those who have a bed in front of a mirror should move it to avoid the soul leaving the physical body and entering the mirror during sleep.

In my family, bedroom doors were always closed when we had company (unless the company was very close relatives or friends), and the reason was for privacy. "No one needs to know how I sleep." It was considered terribly taboo to open a bedroom door that was not yours. Alternatively, there was tremendous curiosity about a person's bedroom configuration because it was very telling, as you can imagine. For instance, a devout churchgoing Roman Catholic widowed grandma's room invariably lacked a mirror, and the foot of the bed was positioned away from the door. The door would be left wide open, to show that she had nothing to hide. However, if she slept facing a mirror with her feet by the door, that bedroom door would always remain closed.

This superstition is an example of one that, in fact, gives instructions, depending on what you want to accomplish. I guess it goes without saying, but I will say it anyway: I sleep facing a mirror with the foot of my bed by the door.

In addition to sleeping position, there is the bedtime routine. Until I grew up and left home, I thought everyone did the exact same routine at bedtime. Maybe you do? Getting ready for bed is very much like getting ready to go somewhere. Wash up and brush teeth. Change into clean pajamas. Comb hair (protective hair style for long hair). Apply some face cream, lip balm, a dab of cologne or perfume. Crack the bedroom window open. Place shoes or slippers beside your bed. Say prayers or meditate. Drink a glass of water. This routine was taught to me when I was very little, and it has its roots in the firm folkloric belief that when we sleep, we "fly off" somewhere. We need to prepare and look presentable. No one took this routine more seriously than my parents.

Now let's get back to dreams and dreaming. Although they can be viewed as all one thing, I have broken down four distinct categories for ease of discussion: dreams, trance, spirit flight, and time travel.

1. Dreams (Passive, Receptive)

Dreams are the involuntary sensory experiences that occur when we are asleep. From a folkloric point of view, they were believed to be communication from the other worlds that came to you while you slept, like a cloud carrying messages that at times would be cryptic and require interpretation and other times be as clear as waking life. The goal with dreaming was to not only remember and interpret them but also to "wake up" in the dream (what is known as lucid dreaming) and be fully aware you are in a dream in order to direct it toward where you want it to go—whether it be to a place or to obtain specific information and outcomes. Because they occur during sleep, it is the involuntary nature that gave dreams more credibility over premonitions or visions, as discussed in the preceding chapter.

If you never or rarely remember your dreams, or if you do not dream, the first thing I recommend is to look at your sleep hygiene. Sleep hygiene consists of a combination of healthy habits and environmental factors that contribute to a good night's sleep. A good night's sleep is conducive to dreaming and beneficial to your overall health. The next thing is to go to sleep with the intention to remember your dreams. This advice sounds simple, and it is, but I admit that I am not very good at remembering to tell myself that I intend to remember my dreams. When I do and I am consistent, I notice a remarkable improvement.

When I am very worried about something, and I remember to remind myself to remember my dreams, I sit for a moment and surrender my worry to my guardian spirit(s) before going to sleep. I envision myself handing over to them a small parcel containing that worry and asking them to hold on to it while I sleep. If I can get over the hurdle of handing it over—it is human nature to hold on tight—I sleep better. I have found the parcel containing the worry is smaller in the morning than it was the night before, and even if I do not remember dreaming, I wake up with a clearer understanding and often a solution. Get into the habit of asking your guardian spirits to help you with solutions to whatever is troubling you. Do the work, and your spirits will come to your aid. You'll get the benefit of a good night's sleep and assistance with your personal matters.

I don't dream every night, or rather, I don't remember my dreams every night. I go through phases when I am totally into my dreams and dreamlife and others when I'm not.

In folk magic, dream work often involves simple but meaningful tools that help us connect with the spirit world, receive messages, and track our inner landscapes. These items support communication with the dead, deepen dream recall, and give structure to the often mysterious language of dreams.

Dream diary or journal paired with a dream dictionary: You can glean a lot of insight from your dreams just by jotting down what you remember upon waking up and combining it with information from a dream dictionary. This is a great start toward the goal of learning your own personal symbolic language. You may find that your meanings are very much in line with common dream dictionary meanings. You may also be surprised at how your personal meanings are completely different and more profound. This is the part of dream work where you work on building your lexicon. My lexicon is an eternal work in progress on the side of my desk, figuratively speaking. I share this information to make the point that you don't need a fully developed personal lexicon to participate in the other activities related to dream work. If you are struggling to remember your dreams, a dream journal is still beneficial. Begin a practice of journaling for a few minutes when you wake up. For example, you can journal about these questions: What emotion are you feeling upon waking up? What was your first thought? Does it feel like you dreamt but do not remember, or does it feel like you had a dreamless sleep?

The most common practice I know is writing a letter to the dead and burning it. After doing so, the dead would respond via dreams or through random conversations with acquaintances or strangers. For example, you write a letter to your beloved dead and burn it. A few days later you are at your local grocery store, and unprompted, the butcher starts a conversation with you on the very subject you wrote about in your letter. During that short exchange, the butcher says something that gives you goosebumps, and you know in your gut that your beloved dead is talking to you.

Spirit mailbox: I don't know if this mailbox has another name. My father called it the mailbox to the dead, which, in his dialect, was a play on the Italian terms for mailbox and coffin. It is a box with a slot where you slip in your letters to the spirits of the dead. Once you slip your letter in, it is now their property, and it is taboo for the sender to retrieve it. It is taboo to open the box for any reason. In the event of the sender's death, the box must be destroyed.

I must share something because I thought I was so clever. When my father was first hospitalized toward the end of his life, per his wishes, I went to his home to retrieve his box to destroy it. I had never seen his spirit mailbox and if I had, it would never have occurred to me what it was. I was expecting a sealed shoe box or something just as mundane. My father was an artist. Of course, his box was a stunning work of art. Destroying it pained me, so I hatched a plan to pry it open, empty and destroy the contents, and keep the box for my use. The blade of the full-tang knife I used to attempt to pry it open snapped off at the slightest pressure, and the blade end that snapped flew toward my face and missed my right eye by mere fractions of an inch, leaving a one-inch cut on my right temple. Spooked (and bleeding a lot as even minor cuts to the head do), I reluctantly tossed the box and the broken knife in a grocery bag and took it where I knew there was a garbage chute that led to an incinerator to dispose of both.

Spirit book: I got the idea to make myself a spirit book from the communication book that was kept on hospital wards for nurses and doctors to leave each other messages related to the ward. In my spirit book, I wrote my messages to the dead, and when I had a dream or a synchronicity following writing that message, I would record the reply from spirit in my book in a different color ink. This spirit book quickly took the place of my dream journal, and I kept it up for years when I lived alone but destroyed it prior to getting married to my first husband. I didn't want to worry about him or anyone else reading it. In hindsight, I could have placed it in a locked box and hidden it, or if I didn't need to have access to it, I could have taken it to my bank and placed it in a safe deposit box.

2. Trance

Trance is an altered state of consciousness in which awareness shifts inward, allowing for deep focus, spiritual connection, or heightened perception. I experience trance a little differently. I often achieve a trance state while being physically engaged in a repetitive task that frees my mind to wander, my body loses awareness of my environment, and my mind feels like being awake in a dream.

I first learned about going into a trance when I was around ten years old. Stories about the fantastic and sometimes prophetic dreams one of my ancestors would have when she spun at her spinning wheel had me completely captivated. Whenever she went to the attic and spun at her spinning wheel, there was no way to get her to stop until she was done because she was in a trancelike state. When she was done, she would descend from the attic with spun wool and news from the other world. How I longed for my very own spinning wheel!

One day, while shelling a bushel of peas my uncle had picked from his garden, I experienced this light trancelike state. All I remember was feeling comfortable and peaceful without any notion of time. That is when I became a little obsessed with any type of repetitive task. I would seek out chores that were repetitive and I could do alone. It was my favorite escape.

The only downside of my little trance obsession as a kid is that ever since then I am prone to involuntarily slip into that space with the slightest repetitive task. That includes engaging in any type of rhythmic or cognitively undemanding activity such as peeling vegetables, walking, commuting as a passenger, or commuting as the driver (this is one where I have to make it a point to remain present because it is not safe!). Also, repetitive sounds such as that of a clock ticking, a metronome, and, of course, a drum. The sound of running water and other white noises. How many people do you know say they do their best thinking and problem-solving in the shower? Perhaps you do too? I experience the most vivid downloads of psychic information and premonitions in the shower. Trance can be voluntary or involuntary.

3. Spirit Flight

Spirit flight, also known as soul journeying, hedge riding, or trance travel, is a key practice in folk witchery and is found in many folk traditions. It refers to the witch's ability to leave the physical body and travel into the spirit world, or different realms of existence. This practice is often used for divining, communicating with spirits, gathering knowledge, or performing magical workings. In medieval and early modern Europe, witches were believed to fly to Sabbats or travel in spirit form to commune with supernatural beings. During the witch trials in medieval Europe, Sabbats were said to be secret gatherings where witches met to worship the devil, cast spells, and take part in wild, forbidden rites. Northeastern Italian folklore describes witches riding winds, animals, or even broomsticks in spiritual form, traveling beyond the mortal world.

To initiate spirit flight, start by creating a protective space, often using tools like protective symbols, salt, or herbs to ensure a safe journey. Ground yourself beforehand with deep breathing or through physical actions like holding or wearing a talisman. As you enter a meditative or trancelike state, visualize or feel your spirit rising above your physical body, guided by your intention. Setting clear intentions is important, whether you're seeking guidance, protection, or answers. Ask for your spirit guide to accompany you and protect you from any unwanted influences, and be respectful of the spirits you may encounter. Once the journey is complete, gently return to your body, grounding yourself by touching the earth or drinking water. As with any magical practice, ensure you maintain clear boundaries and trust in your connection to the spirits that guide you. Always reflect on your experience to deepen your understanding of the spirit realm and your practice.

Benandanti

Any chapter on spirit flight would be incomplete without mentioning the *benandanti*. Their story, preserved through Inquisition records and brought to light by historian Carlo Ginzburg, stands as one of the most vivid and well-documented examples of nocturnal spirit journeys in European folk tradition.

In the northeasternmost region of Italy, particularly in Friuli, healers known as the benandanti were accused of witchcraft in the 16th and 17th centuries. According to local beliefs, babies born with a caul, or "with the shirt" (still covered in the amniotic sac), were destined to become benandanti, healers with protective and spiritual abilities. It was thought that the caul granted them resistance to harm and the power to leave their bodies in spirit form. Their mission was to battle witches and malevolent beings that threatened the fertility of the fields. These night battles occurred during the Ember Days—traditional fasting periods—and saw the benandanti fighting with fennel branches while witches wielded sorghum canes. A benandanti victory meant a prosperous harvest; a loss signified misfortune.

The benandanti were divided into three groups:

Agrarian benandanti: Engaged in spiritual battles for agricultural fertility (mainly men).

Funereal benandanti: Participated in nightly processions, communicating with the dead (mostly women).

Therapeutic benandanti: Practiced healing magic, curing illnesses and wounds, in contrast to the harmful magic of witches (both men and women).

The benandanti were extensively studied by Carlo Ginzburg, whose 1966 work, *The Night Battles*, linked their beliefs to ancient fertility cults and shamanic traditions. Ginzburg argued that inquisitors, initially viewing benandanti as healers, gradually rebranded them as evil devil worshippers. However, historian Franco Nardon, in his 1999 study, challenged Ginzburg's claims. Nardon, analyzing later 17th-century records, found no evidence of a shift in how benandanti were perceived.

Instead, he argued that the Inquisition's focus changed—as fear of the witches' Sabbat declined, some inquisitors forced a connection between benandanti and witches. Despite these efforts, local communities continued to view benandanti as healers and protectors against witchcraft.

Over time, the benandanti's purpose was reframed by outside forces—by inquisitors, shifting fears, and the changing needs of authority. Whether we understand them as folk healers, visionaries, or something more, their story reminds us how easily spiritual work can be misinterpreted or reshaped. I leave it to you to consider what their night battles meant—to them, to those around them, and perhaps even to those who still walk a similar path today.

Sources

Dizionario di eretici, dissidenti e inquisitori nel mondo mediterraneo. A cura di Daniele Santarelli. Edizioni CLORI. Firenze. DOI 10.5281/zenodo.1309444.

Del Col, Andrea. *Benandanti.* In DSI, vol. 1, pp. 172–173.

Ginzburg, Carlo. *I benandanti*. Ricerche sulla stregoneria e sui culti agrari tra Cinquecento e Seicento. Einaudi, Torino, 1966.

Nardon, Franco. *Benandanti e inquisitori nel Friuli del Seicento.* Edizioni dell' Università di Trieste, Trieste, 1999.

Visintin, Dario. *I benandanti e il Sant'Ufficio alla metà del Seicento.* In *Metodi e Ricerche*, n.s., XXVII/1, pp. 23–52.

The Practice of Spirit Flight

Although information about the benandanti dates back at least three hundred years, the practice of night flight or spirit flight for various reasons (such as to battle against opposing forces, to commune with the dead, or to heal the sick) still exists today. I'm going to tell you a secret: Nothing prevents you from doing the same if you feel called to it. No one is going to ask you for proof you were born with a caul. Spirit flight is simple, but it is not easy. It takes practice. Italian immigrants who were so inclined did it all the time and spoke about it openly. It was a common practice to "fly" home to their village in Italy to check on things and visit with loved ones. The following is a recurring experience someone dear to me had; it was always some kind of version of this:

> Last night I dreamt that I went home (their village in Italy). I flew there riding a giant falcon. When I arrived at the town square, everyone was there. Even the dead! There was music and dancing and all the food you can imagine. My late mother was there. She looked so young and beautiful, just like she did when I was a child. She held me in her arms and I could feel her grip and the fabric of her dress and smell the scent of roses in her hair. There was a big fire, and we all danced around it. There were creatures too. Animals and beasts that were half man and half animal. I felt strong. All the pain I normally feel in my left leg was gone. I looked down at my leg and my leg was gone. Then, my mother told me I needed to go home because soon it would be morning. I felt something pulling me from behind and then I began to fall. Falling, falling, falling, and when I hit the ground, I woke up. The first thing I did was look down at my left leg. My leg is there but the pain is gone. I feel lighter today.

I cannot stress enough how normal it was and how open everyone was to talk about their dreams—whether they had a visitation from a dead family member or predictions of future events, or where they went and who they encountered in spirit flight.

Although I broke up the process into components, they are all part of the same whole. I have not yet had an experience as rich as this example, but I am experienced in flight. I will share with you what I know, but please understand that I am a stubborn girl, and I delight in taking things apart to figure out how they work—or rather, how I can make them work for me. This is my recipe for flight:

1. **Invitation:** It begins with something calling me from far away. It's very subtle, but persistent.
2. **Desire:** This seems obvious, but I really need to feel like it.
3. **Need:** This is a sensation I feel in my gut. I need it. There is something there for me, and I need to retrieve it. Or the sensation feels like being "pulled."
4. **Means:** The best way I can describe this is the vehicle I use to fly. It must be something I trust, and it must be something that allows me to suspend disbelief long enough to get off the ground, so to speak.

Here's an example of what I mean by a vehicle to help suspend disbelief:

> I visualize myself and my guardian spirit at the airport. We board the plane. I run through all the things that need to happen for the plane to take off. I feel my body in the seat. I feel the seat belt. I feel the plane taxi down the runway. I feel the plane take off and begin the climb to altitude. Once the plane attains altitude, I wait for the announcement that we can undo our seatbelts. This is when my guardian spirit and I get up from our seats, I climb onto its back, and we fly away from the plane.

Sounds pretty wild, right? A variation of the airplane is quite common among the folk witches I know. With trial and experience, you will find what works for you.

In addition to the preceding steps, certain herbs are believed to assist with spirit flight, often by facilitating altered states of consciousness. However, it's important to approach these herbs with caution, as some can be toxic if not used properly. *Always research thoroughly and consult an expert before using any herbs.* I only feel comfortable including the herbs I use, and you will see from my selection that I am not very adventurous. I take them all in tea form although some can be smoked.

- Chamomile (*Matricaria chamomilla*): Although chamomile is not traditionally considered a primary herb for spirit flight or shamanic journeys in folk magic, it is the primary herb used in Italian folk magic. Chamomile promotes relaxation, aiding in sleep. Easing anxiety can create a conducive environment for lucid dreaming or light astral travel, which are often precursors to spirit flight experiences.

- Mugwort (*Artemisia vulgaris*): This well-known herb is used for enhancing dreams and facilitating visionary experiences. It is often used as a tea or smoked.

- Damiana (*Turnera diffusa*): While best known for its use in sex magic—to heighten sensation and open channels of connection—this plant also plays a role in spirit flight. With mild psychoactive properties, it helps open the mind to spiritual experience. It's often taken as a tea or smoked.

- Lavender (*Lavandula angustifolia*): While primarily known for relaxation, lavender can also aid in meditative and trance-like states. It is often used as a tea and topically as an oil or balm applied to the temples, wrists, or the third eye.

- Blue lotus (*Nymphaea caerulea*): Known for its calming and psychoactive effects, this plant is sometimes used to induce a sense of detachment from the physical world, supporting astral travel.

- Passionflower (*Passiflora incarnata*): Known for its calming effects, this plant can be used to prepare the body and mind for deep meditative states or spirit work.

Remember that herbs should be used in moderation, and it's always best to approach them with respect, following the guidance of experienced practitioners.

5. **Opportunity:** You need time and privacy.

6. **Companion:** I have never intentionally flown alone, meaning without a guardian spirit, but it has happened spontaneously. When it's planned, I always ask a trusted guardian spirit—that is, a winged creature—to accompany me. Having a companion has more to do with my own mental blocks and suspending disbelief because I have had occasions where my guardian spirit was not winged and we still flew.

Simple, right? Yes.
Easy? No. Spirit flight takes practice.

Let me give you some examples based on an airplane as the means of transportation. Sometimes I am just not in the mood to get on a plane. Sometimes my guardian spirit shows up and doesn't have wings. For me to attain flight, I need to be in this space where I am not aware of my physical environment but not asleep, so I need to suspend disbelief. Most times, I fall asleep before arriving at the airport or upon arriving at the airport. Sometimes I get a bad feeling and don't feel safe, so I abort the mission. Sometimes a noise or a sensation in my physical environment shakes me out of it. Sometimes I get shoved back and wake up. Sometimes I have fallen asleep and find myself dreaming something else, but I know I left with my guardian spirit and search the entire dream looking for them to no avail. I have had more involuntary flight experiences since I was very young than successful intentional flight experiences. I suspect the reason has a lot to do with my prejudices about believing in the experiences that happen to me more than the ones I make happen. These experiences typically start out with me running in total darkness in my dream. I am either running from something that is chasing me or running toward something until I run out of ground. Either I run off a cliff, or I trip and start to fall. As I am falling, I think to myself, "Let go. Remember you can fly!" I feel my chest break open and my arms and legs break off, and I have a sensation of what remains of my body floating and rolling like a ball being sucked upward by the base of my spine. The total darkness turns to moonlight. I can see structures and the top of trees. I meet up with the same spirit I always do, and they escort me back home, where I follow them through my bedroom window. Sometimes I wake up immediately. Other times, I land in my bed and fall back asleep.

4. Time Travel

Time travel is a different concept in folk witchery from how it is understood or described in modern science fiction, but many folk traditions involve spiritual time manipulation, glimpses into the past or future, and the ability to step outside linear time. These practices often appear in divination, trance states, dream magic, and spirit flight.

I come from the perspective that time travel is real, but not in the science fiction sense—to my utter dismay. My father was a time traveler, and he indulged in this activity whenever he could. He would be seated in his favorite chair, and his eyes would be open and looking downward and to his left. His lips would be moving as if he were talking, but he wouldn't make a sound. His body remained motionless in the chair. Upon his return, he would describe himself dropping in on past events and experiencing them with all his senses. He knew his triggers and used them to his advantage. Specific scents, tastes, textures, music, art, and so on could instantly fling him back to a specific place in time. He was incredibly psychic and dead-on accurate, especially with his predictions of disaster and misfortune.

A Generation of Time Travelers

I need to make a little side note here: There is no doubt in my mind that this generation that survived World War II and then immigrated all have something not quite right with them, and I mean in the metaphysical sense, not just the effects of the trauma of surviving the war. Who knows what went on that they, terrified and desperate to survive, never spoke about? Which spirits came to their aid, and at what cost? What secrets did they take to their graves?

When I was five years old, I went to live with my aunt (my father's sister) and uncle. Every evening after supper, we would sit outside on the balcony and eat ice cream, and my aunt would tell stories of her youth during World War II. She would describe in vivid detail the sounds of the sirens, planes in the sky, the bombs landing and leaving giant craters where her friends' homes (and often her friends and their family) once were. The smell of "meat roasting" as the livestock burned. I understood they were stories of her experiences and that this all took place in a distant place in a not-so-distant past. Then suddenly, I began to have weird experiences. I would hear an air raid siren and see planes flying overhead. My environment changed in appearance to what I envisioned when my aunt told her stories, and I would run crying to hide under my bed until it was over. After these events, I would say things that I couldn't have known. Things and details my aunt never included in her stories. She told my father about my experiences, and he forbade my aunt from telling any more of those stories in my presence and to not allow me to eat that specific ice cream anymore.

I used to be sure that what I experienced were shocking true stories meeting a child's vivid imagination. My father was certain it was time travel. I wonder if the reality isn't more that we carry our ancestors' memories stored within us. I grew up listening to a lot of stories, family stories about ancestors. These stories were repeated over and over during repetitive tasks, and they would fling me into a space where I felt as if I were there and witnessing them firsthand. These experiences felt so real. I often couldn't tell where or when I was. I felt like I knew the ancestors who were long dead before I was born.

When I do engage in time travel, it is always to the past and to specific places in time and for very short periods of time. Although I won't share all the details with you, my childhood was harsh, and that terrain is a minefield. You may want to keep this in mind if you relate.

Memories are experienced in the mind and can result in some bodily sensations such as feeling warm or sick to one's stomach. We experience time travel with all our senses, which requires us to be in a trance state.

Perfume Time Machine

I have a perfume collection housed in a closed cabinet that I refer to as my time machine. My perfume collection is more than just bottles of fragrance; it is a portal through time, a bridge between past and present. I keep the scents once worn by loved ones who have passed, allowing me to visit them through olfactory time travel. A single breath of their perfume brings back their presence, their essence, as if they are standing beside me once more. When I wear their scent, I feel their spirit drawn close to me, surrounding me in an invisible embrace. The veil between worlds thins, and for a brief moment, we exist together again.

I also have fragrances tied to specific chapters of my own life, each one holding memories and emotions suspended in time. When I wear these scents, I am transported—not just in thought, but in feeling. The emotions, the atmosphere, the sensations of that time wash over me as if I have truly stepped back into that moment. It is more than nostalgia; it is a full-bodied return to the past, where I can relive the joy, sorrow, excitement, or comfort of those days. In my magico-spiritual practice, scent is a powerful tool, not just for remembrance but for connection. Through this ritual, I honor those I have lost, commune with their spirits, and move fluidly between memory, magic, and time itself.

I also do other things to trigger memories or time travel such as preparing certain foods, touching certain textures, exposing myself to specific color palettes, art and making art, makeup, clothing, advertising, books, music, and movies.

It is also important to have a solid present reference to pull me back ASAP when I begin to feel as though I am losing myself. Admittedly, I also have a low tolerance for time travel. As I mentioned earlier, my past is full of land mines, and I can go from having a wonderful experience one moment to needing to get out the next. I have a better tolerance for memories because they are not as immersive, and I can just switch to a different thought.

* * *

I share these experiences with you to make the point that every experience is unique to the individual. It is okay to not know what you are doing and to do it anyway. I share these experiences because my ancestors shared theirs with me, and I am grateful to them and cognizant that you may not have had ancestors who shared these kinds of things with you.

The best thing I ever did for my personal folk magic practice was letting go of the need to find names and labels coined by others for my personal experiences. I highly recommend you do the same. It is very liberating. If you are keen to try some time travel yourself, here are some folk beliefs for you to explore.

Certain places and moments were thought to weaken the boundary between past, present, and future: In European folklore, standing at a crossroads or within a fairy circle at certain times (such as Samhain or Midsummer) could allow glimpses of the past or future. Some legends tell of people entering a cave or a faerie hill and emerging years or centuries later, unaware that time had passed differently for them. Some witches were said to enter deep trances or magical sleep to awaken in a different time, either physically or in spirit.

Many folk magic traditions focus on peering into time rather than physically traveling: using reflective surfaces like black mirrors or water bowls to scry or see visions of the past or future. In the Celtic "Three Drops" method of prophetic vision, drops of sacred water or herbs are placed on the forehead before sleep. Some forms of divination using bones or runes were believed to reveal not just fate but also glimpses of past lives or future events.

Chapter 7

A Guide to Safe and Discreet Practice

Practicing Openly versus Privately

I am going to get right into this topic. Just because all things witchy might appear to be trending and mainstream now (like all trends, it is cyclical, and it's very exciting!), that does not mean it is safe for everyone to be completely open about their witchcraft practice. Just because we engage with a self-selecting group does not mean that there are not other self-selecting groups who are completely opposed to our practices. Never forget that there are still places all over the world where people are put to death for merely being accused and suspected of witchcraft or just for being different from the norm. Just because your partner, friends, and family think it's cool you're a witch, don't assume your professor, employer, clients, children's teachers, family doctor, or anyone who may hold a part of your or your family's fate in their hands feels the same.

I realize the irony of me saying this in my book with my name on it, but I do speak from experience. As you grow older, you gain the confidence to not care about what people think because, as time goes on, fewer and fewer people hold your fate in their hands. The irony is that this confidence and the fact that we become invisible as we age are what permit us to hide in plain sight. Until then, heed my warning and be discerning with who you allow in. Folk magic practitioners have always blended into their cultural and religious communities. It was a matter of survival.

Cultivate Stealth.

If your family and community are religious (and they view anything outside their religion as evil) and your survival depends on your good standing with them, do whatever you need to do to blend in. Attend church. Attend family and community functions. Do what is expected of you until you can be on your own. Once you are on your own, you can relax a little, but when you interact with your family and community, blend in. They do not need to know you don't agree with them. Be smart. Prioritize your needs and safety.

What We Share. What We Don't. Your Spirits Are Yours and Yours Alone.

At this time when it seems everyone is living their lives in front of a camera and posting to social media, I would like to remind you that most of it is a performance. But suppose you are one of those people posting earnestly. I strongly recommend you stop that right now. I too feel that desire to share the things that bring meaning and joy to my life. You don't know who is watching and may be envious and/or wish you harm, and that goes for real life (off the Internet) as well.

I am open to sharing a pretty photo of my altar shrine and examples of spell work, but I do not share images of my working altar or my real magical workings/spells. Just like I do not pray in front of an audience or a camera. If we have company over, all is tucked away from prying eyes.

Keep It Secret. Keep It Sacred.

I learned at the feet of the generation who taught me "Do not tell anyone who your spirits are. They are not for show. They are not playthings or accessories to show off. They are to be respected." The old ones warned against even divulging who your patron saint was for fear that your enemy would send a demon impersonating your patron saint to, at the very least, find out all your secrets or, the very worst, lure you into danger.

Choose your witch community wisely. I have never and will never be a member of a coven because I have always been a solitary creature and folk magic practitioner, so I cannot speak to that experience. Folk witchery is a solitary practice that is enriched by kinship and the sharing of practices and experiences with other trusted practitioners. Be discerning who you open yourself up to. If something or someone doesn't feel quite right, trust your gut. Incidentally, this advice goes for friendships and romantic relationships as well.

Choose your spirit allies wisely. Mind the company you keep. You can never be too careful when it comes to spirits. Take your time and go slow. Beneficent spirits are never pushy. Trickster spirits can be fun when they're helping you out, but you're being tricked too. Pay attention to how these relationships affect your health, mood, life, finances, and relationships with the living. This is a thing, and we need to talk about it.

A Malefic Spirit Is Neither Your Friend nor Your Ally.

Malicious entities may disguise their intentions, pretending to have your best interests at heart, but this is merely deception. Their true nature is one of manipulation, self-interest, and often, destruction. If you find yourself engaging with such a spirit—whether intentionally or by accident—it is crucial to remain vigilant and maintain firm boundaries. These spirits are skilled at exploiting weaknesses, twisting words, and preying on vulnerabilities. They may offer power, knowledge, or assistance, but their aid often comes with hidden costs. Unlike benevolent or neutral spirits, malefic entities do not seek balance or mutual respect. Instead, they operate out of selfish desire, chaos, or outright malice. Some may thrive on fear, conflict, or emotional turmoil, whereas others may attempt to bind or deceive practitioners for their own gain.

You can protect yourself by doing the following: Strengthen your spiritual defenses (through wards, protective charms, or banishing rituals). Never enter agreements lightly because words have power, and spirits can twist intentions. Trust your intuition. If something feels off, it probably is. Maintain control. Never let a spirit dictate terms or demand offerings beyond reason. While some advanced practitioners choose to work with such entities for specific purposes, it is a dangerous path that requires experience, wisdom, and firm spiritual authority. If you are uncertain or unprepared, the best course of action is avoidance and protection. Do not delude yourself that you can control any spirit.

Not all spirits have good intentions, and some may pretend to be helpful while working against you. Whether you are engaging in spirit work, divination, or witchcraft, it's essential to recognize the signs that indicate a spirit may not be an ally.

Signs that your spirit ally may not be right for you:

» The spirit gives conflicting messages. One day, it offers wisdom; the next, it confuses or misleads you. The spirit changes identity, claiming to be one thing but later contradicting itself.

» It makes false promises. It offers power, knowledge, or rewards but never delivers—or demands outrageous things in return.

» The spirit "barges in" on you, demanding constant attention. If a spirit becomes overbearing, demanding contact at all hours, it may be trying to dominate your space. It may try to pressure you into oaths, pacts, or offerings. Exercise extreme caution if it insists on long-term agreements without allowing you to think or refuse.

» It won't leave. A spirit that refuses to leave when asked, or shows up uninvited, is a major bad sign. A true spirit ally respects your free will and personal boundaries.

» Its presence is discomforting or scares you. You feel uneasy in its presence. If something feels not right or unsettling, trust your instincts. The spirit is truthful, but it always shares negative or frightening information. A true ally will be consistent and honest. Be wary of any spirit that seems to manipulate or deceive.

» It makes you feel small. It criticizes you or insults you. It urges you to do things that you are ethically and morally opposed to or things that alienate you from the people who love you. It makes threats or instills fear. Any spirit that claims harm will come to you if you stop working with it is not an ally. Genuine spirit allies operate through mutual respect, not fear or coercion.

Since entering into a relationship with this spirit:

» You experience one misfortune after another.

» You experience ill health. One health problem resolves and another arises.

» You experience exhaustion, a feeling of being drained of your energy.

» (If you read cards) You suddenly cannot read for yourself and/or others, or all your readings are either completely incoherent or always doom and gloom.

» You have a constant feeling of impending doom.

» You suddenly become clumsy and sustain constant physical injuries.

» Although completely healthy, you suddenly develop serious medical problems requiring hospitalization that completely come out of nowhere.

» Unexplained physical disturbances in your environment can indicate an intrusive presence. Objects suddenly move or disappear from where you placed them. You hear whispers, knocks, someone calling out your name (when you are alone), or you see shadowy figures in your peripheral vision. These can be signs of malefic or opportunistic spirits attempting to gain access to you. If you hear someone calling your name and you are alone, do not answer. Wait. If you hear it again, be assertive and say, "Go away." If you hear a knock on your door, confirm that a person is really there before opening your door. If you forget or aren't thinking and open your door, say, "You are not welcome here. Go away." Clap your hands loudly three times and close the door.

» You may experience invasive dreams, intrusive thoughts, or visions. Spirits that appear in dreams without invitation and cause distress should be dealt with cautiously.

This list is not exhaustive, nor is it always caused by a spirit. These are things to keep in mind. Trust your gut. Exercise discernment. If in doubt, seek advice from experienced magicians and occultists you trust.

A magico-spiritual practice is meant to be nourishing and sustaining. It should strengthen and enrich your power, not deplete it.

Recommendations to Keep Your Practice Low-Key or Secret

The following recommendations are just that—recommendations. They are geared toward keeping your practice low-key or secret for the purpose of minding your personal safety. If you are lucky enough that you can practice openly, nothing prevents you from incorporating and customizing these recommendations for yourself.

I have a profound love and appreciation for objects made of natural materials that are handcrafted, rustic, and organic looking in natural colors, plus tactile, simple, elegant, restrained, and timeless. I am also a huge fan of objects that are multipurpose. Witchcraft is an art, and personal aesthetic matters to make us feel good in our magical skin.

Personal aesthetic matters on so many levels. For privacy, matching your magical tools to your personal aesthetic does most of the work of blending them into your environment, hidden in plain sight. Here is an example to better illustrate what I mean. If your personal aesthetic is athletic, for your magical practice and tools to hide in plain sight, they should blend in with that aesthetic. Some of my earliest magical tools were a baseball and a catcher's mitt and a hockey stick. If you play Dungeons & Dragons, I cannot think of a better cover to hide a true magical practice in plain sight.

When I first got into witchcraft in the mid-eighties, there was very little information available to a teenager with no money. Most of my information was bits and pieces from library books (nonfiction and fiction), movies, television, and whatever information I could get from the occult-oriented people I knew. I owned a deck of playing cards, a deck of tarot cards, and one book on witchcraft in the Italian language. I kept notes in a binder, but it was only on information I gathered. Even that was scant because I was young and had a memory like a steel trap and therefore didn't feel the need to write anything down. On the one hand, I wish I had kept a journal of what I did. The spells I cast. The things I experimented with. What the results were. Dreams. Synchronicities. Freaky occurrences with spirits, including Ouija board experiences. But, on the other hand, I am glad that I didn't because later I had someone in my life who, if they had gotten their hands on it, would have used it against me. That is something to consider if you are on the fence about keeping a magic book.

Grimoire

A folk magic grimoire is a personal book of spells, rituals, and knowledge. I prefer my grimoire to be a record of what I have already done—not theory, not intention, but practice. I only write down spells and rituals that I've tried and found to be effective. Like I do with a recipe book, I return to them whenever I need to repeat or adapt them. And just like with recipes, having a record of what's worked lets me adjust it for different situations. I can refer back to what worked and adjust it to suit a different purpose. Keep your grimoire simple, practical, and deeply connected to your practice, culture, and surroundings.

Here are some suggestions on ways to structure and organize your grimoire. You can choose to divide one book into different sections, or you can have multiple journals, each one dedicated to a topic, or a combination of both. Like I said, these are suggestions to help you experiment and figure out what works for you. Be open to changing your mind and your system. I have lost count of how many times I have changed mine!

To set up your grimoire, begin by including sections based on natural cycles and timing, such as moon phases and magic, seasonal traditions, and weather-based elemental magic. Add details about local and cultural practices, including sacred plants, herbs, stones, bones, shells, and animal omens. Record your divination methods, dream symbols, and spirit work, such as communicating with ancestors or land spirits. Include a section for spells and rituals, such as protection, healing, fertility, and banishing. Dedicate a part to personal magic and notes, where you can record your experiences, successful spells, and insights. You may also want to have a separate journal dedicated specifically to your spirits and deities, where you can document interactions, offerings, and guidance. Use a physical book, binder, or digital format, and write in your own words to make the grimoire personal and adaptable. Keep an open mind and let your grimoire evolve with your practice. The format you choose will depend on many factors. Now that we've got the technical stuff out of the way, we can move on to the fun stuff!

Thrift stores are my favorite place to shop for ordinary stuff that can be upcycled into witchcraft tools and supplies. Thrift a hardcover book and turn it into a grimoire with secret compartments. If you like your grimoire to be a large book, old technical textbooks work well for this purpose. Match it to your studies or interests, and you just scored bonus invisibility points. You can cut the pages out of the book and use the cover to conceal your grimoire. You can keep the pages in the textbook and cover them with gesso. You can then create grimoire pages interspersed with the textbook pages. Other types of books that I think make great grimoires are old photo albums. I especially love the really old leather-bound ones with black pages. I have a few two-page spreads of black paper in my grimoire that I use as void space to look into when I meditate. My local thrift stores are always stocked with obsolete office and electronics accessories. Look for things like binders that zip shut, calendar or planner covers, or (my favorite) yellowed loose-leaf or college-ruled paper. As a matter of fact, you can score a lot of paper for cheap and then stain it with tea or coffee if you like. Also, check out craft supplies, home décor, and fashion accessories for embellishments.

If you relish the thought of one day leaving behind a grimoire full of secret information that *can* be decoded, write in a different language.

If you speak a language other than what everyone around you does, even if you just learned it at school, write it in that language. If you would rather leave behind a grimoire that *cannot* be decoded, write in that foreign language and combine the language with a type of secret language. Other options are using symbols or making up your own language. All that matters, honestly, is that *you* can read it. Imagine going through all that effort, and when you return days/weeks/months/years later to read something in your grimoire, even you don't know what you're looking at. Yeah, I've done that. If you want to be even more secretive, go digital—password-protected on your mobile device, laptop, desktop. For ultimate portability, store your grimoire on a thumb drive. Wear the thumb drive as an amulet for protection or a talisman for good luck!

Some witches choose to create stunningly beautiful elaborate journals (also called Book of Shadows) simply for the pleasure of the artistic process. I fall somewhere in the middle. I do create art in my grimoire, but what I am really keen on is keeping a working record of my magical shenanigans. My grimoire is a place that holds recipes for oils and incenses I have concocted and spells I have cast that were successful—a place to record thoughts and observations related to my spell work. My grimoire is my sacred space that contains two-page-spread shrines dedicated to specific purposes, and two-page altar spaces where I perform my spells and rituals. Once completed, my magical workings are concealed by artwork glued over them, and only I know what magic resides underneath.

What do I mean when I say I conceal spells and magical workings in my grimoire? Years ago, I did a working and wrote it in my grimoire, as I always do. This one was so deeply personal that seeing it in my grimoire made me feel exposed and vulnerable. Even more so at the thought of anyone else seeing it. I felt exposed. I thought about ripping out the pages and burning them, but that did not feel right. I thought about covering it up and that felt better. I covered the two-page spread with artwork, prayers, poetry, and embellishments that symbolized what the spell was for and the spirit I had asked for help. I turned that two-page spread into a shrine to that specific spirit and purpose. Nowadays, I will visit that two-page spread and mist it with the appropriate fragrance as an offering of love and ongoing gratitude to that spirit.

Commonplace Book

I don't see the value in filling my grimoire with information directly copied from books I own. I do, however, see the value in keeping a commonplace book in addition to a grimoire. A commonplace book is essentially a personal collection of notes and ideas from books, articles, and other sources. Instead of just copying word for word from your references, you record information in your own words, organizing it by subject or theme. This method makes it easier to access and reflect on the material when you need it. A commonplace book serves as a tool for recording your thoughts, insights, and research, creating a system that helps you organize the knowledge you've gathered in a way that is meaningful and useful to you.

Sacred Space

You don't have to have an altar, but many folk witches maintain an altar (or more than one) to have a sacred space to honor and commune with their spirits and as a place for magical work. Folk magic altars vary widely depending on culture, tradition, and purpose. They often serve as sacred spaces for honoring spirits, deities, and ancestors, or performing magic. First, I want to describe some typical altars specific to folk magic practices. Ways to make them low-key or secret will follow. These examples are from different folk magic traditions:

> **Protective home altar:** This altar is set up for the purpose of household protection (honoring house spirits), banishing negativity, and spiritual cleansing. This type of altar is commonly seen in Italian folk magic, folk Catholicism, and Pennsylvania Dutch Hexerei. Its purpose is warding off evil, blessing the home, and keeping away negative forces. To set up your ancestral altar, you may include protective symbols that hold personal meaning, such as crosses, pentagrams, or other sacred symbols. Items like holy water, holy oil, and blessed salt can be used for purification and blessings. Candles, particularly black for banishing and white for protection, help set

the spiritual atmosphere. Iron objects, such as nails, horseshoes, or railroad spikes, are traditionally used for their protective qualities. Bundles of protective plants like rue (*Ruta graveolens*), snakeroot (*Bistorta officinalis*), and blackthorn (*Prunus spinosa*) can serve as additional safeguards. To absorb negativity, a bowl of salt, vinegar, or eggshell powder may be placed on the altar. Most importantly, incorporate personal mementos and keepsakes—items that bring you comfort and connection in your spiritual practice.

Ancestral altar: This altar is set up for the purpose of honoring the dead. This type of altar is commonly seen in Italian folk magic, hoodoo, Mexican folk magic, and other European traditions. Its purpose is to have a sacred space to honor ancestors, seek guidance, and offer respect. Your ancestral altar is a designated space where you can engage in spirit communication with your ancestors for the purpose of asking for their guidance and protection. When setting up an ancestral altar, you may include photographs of your ancestors, along with personal heirlooms or keepsakes that once belonged to them. Offerings such as food, coffee, alcohol, tobacco, flowers, and perfume can be placed on the altar to honor their memory. Candles, either white or in colors significant to your ancestry, provide light and spiritual presence. Incense, such as copal, myrrh, or frankincense, is commonly used, though this may vary depending on your ancestral traditions. Some practitioners also include earth or graveyard dirt taken specifically from an ancestor's grave. Most importantly, your altar should feature personal mementos and keepsakes that foster a deep sense of connection with your ancestors.

Conjure altar: This altar is set up for the purpose of rootwork and spirit work aimed at protection, prosperity, love spells, and spiritual guidance. This type of altar is commonly seen in hoodoo, conjure, and Southern American folk magic. Its purpose is for working with spirits, saints, and ancestors, and performing rootwork. When setting up a conjure altar, you may include a Bible or a Psalms book, often left open to specific verses for spiritual guidance. A glass of water is commonly placed on the altar to aid in spirit communication. Dirt from crossroads or a graveyard may be used for its symbolic and magical significance. Mojo bags or gris-gris—small spell bags filled with items for protection, love, or luck—are often included as well. Saint candles—tall, cylindrical glass-encased candles featuring images of saints and corresponding prayers—can be lit for divine assistance. Specially crafted oils for purposes such as money drawing, fast luck, or love are also commonly used. Most importantly, your altar should reflect your personal connection to the practice, so include objects that resonate with you and feel meaningful in your spiritual work.

Genii locorum (local spirits) altar: This altar is set up for the purpose of honoring the protective spirits of place such as local spirits, nature deities, and fae beings. It is set up as a sacred space to connect with nature spirits and perform fae magic and land blessings. This type of altar is commonly seen in Celtic folk magic, northern Italian and Slavic folk magic, and Appalachian folk traditions. To set up a genii locorum altar, you may include offerings such as fresh water, honey, milk, and wine to honor the spirits of the land. Natural elements like fresh flowers, twigs, acorns, feathers, and pretty stones help establish a connection with the surrounding environment. Shiny coins or bells can be placed on the altar to attract good spirits. Candles in green or white are commonly used, though brown can also be a meaningful choice if available. Most importantly, your altar should reflect your personal connection to the land, so include mementos and keepsakes that feel sacred to you and align with your practice.

These are just some examples of folk magic altars and some common items that are used to set them up. The goal is to create an altar that reflects your spiritual beliefs and magical practice. I also want to add that your altar is not static: Your altar(s) will change and evolve as your practice changes and evolves.

When creating your own folk magic altar, consider who or what you are honoring, such as spirits, ancestors, deities, or nature. Choose appropriate tools and offerings based on your focus. Decide where to place your altar, whether in a private space or a central location within your home. Finally, plan how to keep your altar active, whether through making regular offerings, lighting candles, or performing prayers.

If you want an altar and you want to keep it low-key, completely private, or even portable, there are many options. You can create an altar or shrine in your grimoire. Create art, glue things on a page, create a two-page spread that you open, and use that surface to do magical workings. You can make a portable altar in a box, bag, or binder that doesn't look like much of anything on the outside. When it is not in use, close it up and put it away. If you sew, you can create a cloth that closes like a book and the inside has all the items important to you pinned, glued, or sewn on. You can create a password-protected altar or shrine on your smartphone, tablet, personal computer, or within a video game. Photos and photo albums of ancestors go basically unnoticed.

Pick a place and make it your sacred space. It can be anywhere. A room in your home. A chair. The inside of a closet. A blanket fort. Your balcony. Your backyard/garden. A tree. A pond. A park. A bus stop. Your car. The public library. Graveyard. Church. Animal sanctuary. The woods. A favorite tree. Anywhere that feels sacred to you is sacred space. You can have multiple sacred spaces. A favorite coffee shop or restaurant. Your sacred space can easily be adapted to your personal level of physical mobility. You can create whatever mood you need with videos of fire burning in a fireplace, sounds of rain or the forest, and so on. Your favorite picture or coffee-table book can be your sacred space. And, of course, your mind. You can create a sacred space where you have an altar in your mind and go to that place in meditation whenever you want to. If, however, visualization is not your strength, or your brain is just not wired that way, then the sacred space and altar in a book or in a box that you can spend time visiting serves the exact same purpose.

Folk Divination Using Common Objects

Folk divination is deeply connected to everyday life, relying on natural signs, simple tools, and traditional methods passed down through generations. It is practical, accessible, and adaptable to any lifestyle. Observing animal behavior, monitoring weather patterns, or using household items for divination can provide insight without drawing attention.

If you prefer to keep your divination practice discreet, playing cards are an excellent alternative to tarot; they are so common that they raise no suspicion. You can even assign tarot meanings to a standard deck of playing cards. Other subtle divination tools include herbal information cards, flashcards, nonwitchcraft books for bibliomancy, and Scrabble or Bananagrams tiles in place of runes or a spirit board. Any pendant on a string can function as a pendulum.

To begin incorporating folk divination discreetly into your practice, start with simple, accessible methods such as reading candle flames, interpreting tea leaves, or paying attention to dreams. Keeping a divination journal can help track patterns, signs, and omens over time. You may also explore natural elements like water, fire, bones, stones, dried beans, or leaves—materials that may hold ancestral connections.

Developing skill in divination, like any psychic ability, requires patience and practice. Don't be discouraged if the results aren't immediate. Think of your intuitive psychic ability as a muscle. The more you experiment and refine your methods, the stronger your intuitive abilities will become. Folk divination is meant to be flexible. Adapt it to suit your personal style and spiritual path.

Curios and Charms

Curios are natural or symbolic objects used in folk magic for their spiritual and magical properties. They can be minerals, bones, charms, or everyday items believed to hold power. Depending on tradition, they are often used for protection, love, luck, and banishing magic. Curios can be worn as jewelry or carried in pockets, mojo bags, or pouches. Or they can be placed on altars as offerings or sources of power. You also can hang them on doors or walls for protection and blessings.

Common curios in folk magic include natural items such as feathers, bones, rocks, seashells, plant seeds, acorns, pine cones, twigs, tree bark, dried leaves, and plant roots. Handmade and enchanted objects include beads, dolls, or plushies filled with dried herbs, flowers, and stones that are magically charged. Folk magic practitioners often wear discreet yet powerful amulets for protection, luck, and spiritual strength. These pieces of jewelry are believed to ward off negativity, attract blessings, and serve as personal talismans.

Popular Protective Amulets and Their Meanings

Folk magic practitioners use protective jewelry in several ways. It is often worn daily for continuous protection and can be enchanted with prayers, spells, or anointing oils. Some practitioners give protective jewelry to loved ones as a safeguard. These items can be placed under pillows or near entryways for added protection. Many also personalize their jewelry by carving symbols, anointing it with herbs or oils, charging it under the moon or sun, or dedicating it to a specific deity. These amulets serve as both spiritual tools and meaningful adornments. Curios are a simple yet powerful way to infuse magic into everyday life. Whether found, crafted, or inherited, they serve as meaningful tools in personal and ancestral folk traditions.

- Nazar (evil eye) amulet: A blue eye-shaped charm that protects against the evil eye and negative energy.
- Cornicello (Italian horn): A twisted horn-shaped amulet from Italian folk magic that brings luck and protection.
- Hamsa hand (Hand of Fatima/Miriam): A hand-shaped charm that shields against harm and brings good fortune.
- Mano fico (fig hand): A closed fist with a thumb between the fingers, used for warding off curses and envy.
- Mano cornuto (horned hand): A hand-gesture-shaped talisman for protection, especially against the evil eye.
- Triquetra (Celtic knot): A triple-knot symbol representing protection, unity, and the cycles of life.
- Serpent jewelry: Worn for spiritual protection, the serpent represents wisdom, healing, and deep change—both transformation and transmutation.
- Animal talismans: Pendants featuring animals such as owls (wisdom), wolves (protection), or ravens (foresight) for spiritual strength.

Amber and jet: A traditional pairing in many folk traditions, worn as beads or pendants sometimes made into prayer beads and rosaries. Amber, long used in Slavic traditions, brings beauty, healing, harmony, and protection. Jet acts as a purifier, drawing out unwanted energy while welcoming in the good. The Romans believed jet protected against evil spirits and the evil eye.

Any jewelry can be used for magical intent. It doesn't have to be traditional or obviously spiritual. What matters is the meaning and energy you give it. Rings, bracelets, necklaces, and even earrings can be quietly charged with protection, blessing, or other intentions. Charging jewelry is especially useful when you want to keep your folk magic practice low-key or private. Magic doesn't need to be seen or be obvious to be powerful.

Spirit Mailbox

As I mentioned in chapter 6, a spirit mailbox is a sacred container used in folk magic to hold written letters, petitions, or offerings for spirits, ancestors, or deities. Practitioners write their requests, prayers, or intentions on paper and place them inside. I just place paper in mine, but other practitioners I know often place items that are symbolic to their personal practice and purpose. The spirit mailbox is made of wood, and it serves as a conduit for communication, allowing the message to be delivered to the spirit world. My box only has a slot going in. Once in, the letters never come out. I write my letter, conduct my ritual, and then place the letter in the box. If the box is full, it must be burned.

I would not own a spirit mailbox if I were practicing on the down-low because I would always be worried about it being discovered. However, I would instead look for a ceramic piggy bank, preferably the kind that does not have an opening on the bottom. If the only one I could find had an opening on the bottom, I would just glue that opening shut.

I have even used the Recycle Bin on my desktop. Write my digital letter to the dead. Conduct my ritual. Pop it in the Recycle Bin. Empty Recycle Bin. Done. I have also written my note to the dead and then passed it through a shredder. Burning is always a great option, provided you can do it safely, but it is not necessary.

Incense/Oils

If you can't use incense, for whatever reason, there are effective smoke-free alternatives. Many folk traditions already use herbs, water, sound, and light for the same purposes as the burning of incense. Herbal sachets and charm bags can be made of cloth and filled with dried herbs for cleansing, protection, or attraction. I like a combination of rue, lavender, and rosemary for peace and protection.

You can simmer herbs, citrus peels, and spices in a pot of water to release their energy. My favorites are cinnamon, orange peel, and bay leaves for prosperity and protection. Alternatively, you can steep herbs in hot water, strain, and use the infused water as a spiritual wash or room spray. My favorite is rose.

Another option is the use of sound. Banging on pots and pans and ringing brass bells are methods used in European folk magic to ward off spirits. You also can whistle and clap hands through rooms and doorways to cast out unwanted spirits. Or you can sprinkle or mist Florida water or other spiritual colognes.

Candles

Some alternatives to burning candles are LED lights, battery-operated candles (I love the ones that flicker like a real candle), and wax melts (I carve symbols into the wax melt before placing in wax warmer).

Creating and Accessing Your Inner Sacred Space

If meditation and visualization come naturally to you, make the most of these abilities by building a rich inner world—a sacred space within your mind where you can store wisdom, tools, and spiritual energy. Imagine a special room or sanctuary in your mind or on the astral plane, a place you can return to whenever you need guidance, strength, or clarity. Guided meditations or journeying exercises can be especially useful in helping you access this space. Simply put on your earbuds, relax, and let the audio lead you there.

If creating a sacred space doesn't come easily at first, don't be discouraged! Like any skill, it takes time and practice to strengthen your ability to visualize and connect with your inner sanctuary. Start small, be patient with yourself, and trust that, with consistency, your sacred space will become clearer and easier to access.

Witchcraft for Others

Folk witches historically served their communities as healers, diviners, and protectors, using herbal remedies, charms, and spells to address illness, misfortune, and spiritual concerns. They performed love magic, fertility rites, and weather workings, ensuring prosperity and wellbeing. Many acted as mediators with spirits or ancestors, offering guidance through divination and dream interpretation. In times of crisis, they provided curse-breaking, protection, and justice magic. Despite suspicion from authorities, they were often trusted figures, blending practical knowledge with mystical insight to support their neighbors.

Should you cast spells on behalf of others? This is a personal choice that each practitioner must make for themselves. It's not my place to dictate what you should or shouldn't do. Everyone is free to follow their own path. My goal is simply to share my thoughts and insights from years of practice.

Putting yourself out there requires you to have a thick skin. You are providing quite a sought-after service, yet it is still taboo. You may be maligned. You may be ridiculed. There are people who will wish you harm either because your craft goes against their beliefs, or they are insecure and envious of you or are in competition with you.

Know what you are getting into. This is a tough one for me. I have had experiences where I thought I knew what I was getting into and then learned that I did not have all the information to make an informed decision as to whether to help or not. Nowadays, if it is a request for something super straightforward like diagnosing and dispelling the evil eye, I am perfectly okay with that. In the case of defensive magic for someone near and dear to me, that too I am perfectly okay with. Where I draw the line is that I do not cast spells of any kind on behalf of other people. The reason is that there is no way to really know the truth of whatever is truly going on with the requester and the target. There is no way to ever know the heart of the person requesting the service, and there is certainly no way of knowing the heart of the target of the spell. Therefore, I do not engage in any of these scenarios. All magic comes at some kind of cost, and I never want to place myself in a position where I (and all I hold dear) can potentially be spiritually harmed in the crossfire.

Be honest about your skill level. Doing so is not only ethical but also keeps you safe. It is human nature to want to help others, but if you engage in magic that is way above your skill level without the help of an experienced mentor, you can easily find yourself in over your head, and suddenly both you and the person requesting the service are in trouble.

Know your worth and value what you offer. Whether you are charging money, bartering, or doing it for free, your skill, time, and effort have value. Maintain your boundaries, and a little word to the wise: Even if you don't want to or feel weird about it, charge something. It is a sad but true fact that people value what they pay for more than what they get for free. Charging also prevents you from being used and exploited.

If you're considering offering your services, it is helpful to set clear boundaries on the types of services you offer to manage clients' expectations. Know the laws in your area and make sure you post the requisite disclaimers. Charge fair prices to value your time and skill. Screen clients and remember that you have the right to decline your services if something does not feel right. Maintain privacy if you are concerned about your safety.

Chapter 8

Common Folk Magic Spells from Around the World

Folk magic traditions from around the world share many common spells, reflecting universal human needs and concerns. Here, we'll look at some of the most common types of spells found in cultural folk magic globally.

1. Protection Spells

Evil Eye Protection Spell Using Red Thread

(Mediterranean, Middle East, Americas, Asia, Europe)

The thread is typically made of red wool or cotton and is worn around the wrist or ankle, or tied or stitched onto clothing. In many traditions, the thread must be gifted or blessed by a trusted elder, spiritual figure, or a family member for it to be effective. Some practitioners anoint it with protective oils, recite prayers, or knot it while speaking intentions of protection. Once worn, the thread acts as a barrier against negative energy and is usually kept on until it naturally falls off or breaks, at which point it is discarded and replaced with a new thread if needed.

Salt and Water Purification Spell

(Worldwide)

Salt's natural preservative and purifying qualities have made it a powerful symbol and tool across many cultures and spiritual traditions. Salt and water are used to cleanse spaces and ward off negativity. To perform a salt and water purification spell, dissolve a pinch of salt in a bowl of clean water. Speak a prayer, chant, or blessing while stirring clockwise, all the while focusing on your intent to cleanse and protect. This ritual clears negative energy and strengthens spiritual boundaries. Sprinkle the water around your home, workspace, or altar, or use it to anoint doorways, windows, and yourself for protection. When I make mine with fresh tap or spring water, I use what I need and discard the rest. To keep some on hand stored in a glass bottle, I boil the water for five minutes, leave it to cool, and then perform the spell with the salt. Boiling the water for five minutes makes it shelf stable and prevents the growth of microorganisms.

Iron for Protection

(Europe, Africa, Asia, Americas)

Iron is used in protection spells to repel evil spirits and bad luck. Take an iron object, such as a nail, horseshoe, or railroad spike, and hold it in your hands while focusing on your intent for protection. Bury iron nails at the four corners of your home or property to create a protective barrier. Hang a horseshoe above your doorway, open end up, to catch and hold good luck while repelling negativity. Carry a small iron charm in your pocket or wear iron jewelry for personal protection. To strengthen its power, periodically cleanse the iron with salt water or smoke from protective herbs like rosemary or cedar.

2. Love and Attraction Spells

Honey Jars and Sweetening Spells

(Americas, Caribbean, Europe)

The purpose of a love spell is to attract love or make someone favor you. Write the name of your desired person on a small piece of paper, along with words of intention (such as love, kindness, or reconciliation). Fold the paper toward you and place it in a small, clean jar. Add enough honey to cover the paper, along with sweet herbs like cinnamon or rose petals for extra attraction. Seal the jar and shake it gently while focusing on your intention. Light a pink or red candle on top of the jar, letting the wax drip down as you visualize love and harmony growing. Repeat as needed, keeping the jar hidden in a safe place.

Herbal and Floral Charms

(Asia, Middle East, Europe, Africa, Americas)

Rose, jasmine, or apple-based charms are used for love and attraction. Select love-drawing herbs such as dried rose petals, jasmine flowers, or apple blossoms. Place them in a small cloth pouch or a locket if you happen to have one. As you assemble the charm, focus on your intention, whispering words of love or desire. Carry the charm with you, tuck it under your pillow, or wear it close to your heart to draw love and affection into your life. Refresh the herbs as needed to maintain their potency.

Binding Love Spell

(Various Traditions Worldwide)

These spells used to secure love often involve knots, red thread, or personal items. Take a red thread, ribbon, or cord and two taglocks (personal items)—such as photos, names written on paper, hair, nail clippings, or bodily fluids, belonging to you and your desired partner.

As you tie the thread around the items, focus on your intention, reciting a love-focused incantation. Knot the thread securely, visualizing the bond strengthening between you both. Store the bound items in a safe place, such as under your bed or in a special box. Always perform love bindings with care, ensuring they align with your ethical beliefs.

3. Money and Prosperity Spells

Coin and Rice Offerings

(Asia, West Africa, Latin America)

To perform this ritual to attract abundance and prosperity, place uncooked rice in a bowl and scatter coins on top, symbolizing wealth. Focus on your intention for prosperity and abundance as you prepare the offering. You can enhance the ritual by lighting incense or candles and offering a prayer or wish. After a few days, dispose of the offering by burying it or placing it in an area symbolizing abundance, like a garden or near water. This ritual invites positive energy and financial growth into your life.

Bay Leaf and Cinnamon Spells

(Europe, North Africa, Middle East, South Asia, Americas)

To perform this spell for prosperity and success, write your specific desire for prosperity or success on a bay leaf. Sprinkle cinnamon powder on the leaf to enhance the power of your intention. Hold the leaf in your hands while focusing on your goal; then burn the bay leaf safely, allowing the smoke to carry your intention into the spirit world. Alternatively, you can place the bay leaf and cinnamon in a jar or pouch and carry it with you as a charm to draw success and financial abundance.

Fast Luck Mojo Bags

(Southern United States, Caribbean)

To create one of these mojo bags for attracting quick good fortune, place a lodestone, pyrite, or High John the Conqueror root into a small cloth bag. Each item is known for its specific magical properties: Lodestone attracts positive energy, pyrite brings prosperity, and High John the Conqueror root is renowned for success and victory. As you fill the bag, focus on your intention for fast luck. Once it is assembled, carry the mojo bag with you, keeping it close for continued good fortune, and periodically recharge it with your energy or by anointing it with oils or herbs.

4. Healing Spells

Egg Cleansing

(Southern Europe, Latin America, Caribbean)

This folk practice is used to remove illness and negative energy. To perform the cleansing, take a raw egg and pass it over the body in a smooth, circular motion, starting from the head and moving downward. As you do so, focus on the intention of removing negativity. After the egg has been passed over the body, crack it into a glass of water and observe the results. The way the egg appears—such as the shape of the yolk or bubbles—can indicate the type of energy or illness being removed. Dispose of the egg and water outside if possible or flush down the toilet, to release the negativity.

Herbal Healing Charms

(Worldwide)

These charms are used in folk magic across various cultures to promote healing and restore balance. Commonly used herbs include chamomile for relaxation, garlic for protection and purification, and rosemary for mental clarity and to support the grieving process. To create a healing charm, bundle the herbs together, tie them with a natural string or thread, and hang them near your bed or in a place where healing energy is needed. You can also carry the charm with you or place it under your pillow for restful sleep. The herbs' medicinal properties combined with the intention of healing help support the body and spirit.

Prayer and Candle Healing Rituals

(Latin America, Caribbean, Southern Europe, Philippines, North America, Central and West Africa)

Common in Catholic-influenced folk magic, these rituals involve lighting candles, often in specific colors, while reciting prayers or invoking saints for healing. For example, a white candle may be used for purity and protection, while a green candle could be used for health. As you light the candle, focus your intention on healing, and say prayers and blessings or incantations aloud, asking for divine assistance. The light of the candle symbolizes the presence of spiritual energy, while the prayer strengthens the connection to the divine and guides the healing process.

5. Banishing and Curse Removal Spells

Smoke Cleansing

(Worldwide)

Smoke cleansing rituals are practiced around the world and often used for banishing, protection, and curse removal. These rituals involve burning plant material, incense, or resin and allowing the smoke to carry your intention. To perform these spells, light sacred herbs and/or resins. Allow the smoke to rise and pass the smoke over yourself, a space, or an object to clear away negative energy and harmful influences. The act is both physical and spiritual: The smoke becomes a medium for purification, a way to call in protection, and a signal to unseen forces that you are claiming the space for healing and safety.

Uncrossing Spells

(Latin America, Caribbean, Southern United States, Southern Europe, West and Central Africa, Philippines)

This kind of uncrossing spell is a global practice with local flavor. What changes are the specific herbs, prayers, or cultural frameworks, but the intention is the same: to remove harm and restore spiritual balance. To perform an uncrossing, you can take a spiritual bath with ingredients like salt, basil (Lamiaceae family), rosemary (*Salvia rosmarinus*), or crushed eggshells, which are believed to clear negative energy. Another method involves lighting candles (often black for banishing or white for protection) and using herbs or oils like fiery wall of protection oil to help remove hexes or jinxes. As you perform the ritual, focus on breaking the hold of the curse or bad luck and ask for healing and protection to restore balance in your life.

Mirror Reversal Spells

(Worldwide)

These spells are used to reflect negativity, curses, or harmful intentions back to their sender. Typically, a mirror is placed facing outward, sometimes with protective herbs or oils around it, to reflect any malevolent energy away from the practitioner (or, by the practitioner on behalf of a target). In some practices, the practitioner may visualize the curse being reversed, while others may write the name of the person sending the negative energy on a piece of paper and place it behind the mirror. This type of spell is meant to send the harmful intentions back, neutralizing their effect and returning the harmful intentions to their source.

6. Divination and Spirit Communication Spells

Pendulums and Bone Throwing
(Worldwide)

Divination practices involving pendulums and bone throwing (or similar object casting) are found worldwide. While the specific methods and cultural meanings vary, the core idea of using objects to seek guidance from spiritual or unseen realms is a nearly universal aspect of folk magic and shamanic traditions across many continents and cultures. These spells are used to receive guidance and communicate with spirits. In pendulum divination, a practitioner holds a pendulum over a surface, asking yes-or-no questions or seeking guidance on a specific issue. The pendulum's movement is interpreted as a response. Bone throwing involves tossing bones, stones, or similar objects onto the ground and interpreting their positions and patterns to gain insight. Both methods rely on intuitive interpretation and are often used to seek answers from spiritual realms or to receive guidance in decision-making.

Dream Magic and Mugwort Tea
(Europe, East Asia, Americas)

The purpose of this spell is to induce prophetic dreams and enhance spirit communication. Mugwort, an herb known for its dream-enhancing properties, is commonly brewed into tea before bedtime to promote vivid dreams and facilitate a deeper connection with the spiritual realm. To use this method, simply steep a teaspoon of dried mugwort in hot water for about 10 to 15 minutes and drink it before sleep. This tea can help you unlock intuitive messages, receive spiritual guidance, and experience dreams that offer insight into future events or personal challenges.

Spirit Offerings
(Worldwide)

To honor and communicate with spirits, offerings such as candles, food, or tobacco are presented as a gesture of respect and to invite spiritual guidance or protection. To perform a spirit offering, place your chosen items on an altar or sacred space dedicated to the spirits you wish to honor. Light a candle to symbolize illumination and spiritual connection, offer food or drink as a sign of gratitude, and use tobacco or incense as a way to invite the spirits to communicate. This ritual is believed to strengthen bonds with ancestors and invite blessings into your life.

7. Weather and Nature Magic

Rain-Calling Rituals
(Americas, Africa, Asia, Oceania, Australia)

To summon rain during times of drought or to ensure a good harvest, stand barefoot outdoors in an open space, grounding yourself to the earth. Raise your arms above your head, palms open to the sky, and close your eyes to center your energy. Begin by visualizing the rain with all five senses: See the dark clouds gathering, feel the cool droplets on your skin, hear the soft patter of raindrops, smell the fresh scent of rain on the earth, and taste the moisture in the air. Focus on feeling the rain soaking the land and imagine it nourishing the soil. Call out to the spirits of water and air, asking for their help in bringing rain. Hold this visualization for as long as you can; then express gratitude for the rain you're calling forth, trusting the natural forces to respond. Alternatively, create an altar with natural elements like water, stones, or plants. Use a drum, rattle, or chant to invoke the spirits of water, air, and earth, while focusing on your intention for rain. You may also use offerings like tobacco, food, or herbs to appease the spirits. In some traditions, practitioners dance or move rhythmically to mimic the falling rain, aligning their energy with the forces of nature. Rain-calling rituals are performed to encourage the rain to come and restore balance to the land.

Wind Spells with Whistling or Knots

(Europe)

Specifically, these wind spells are found within Celtic, Norse, Northeastern Italian, and Slavic folk traditions. These spells are used to manifest change. To perform a wind spell, begin by standing outside in an open area, where the wind can be felt. If using whistling, take a deep breath and whistle into the wind, asking it to bring about the change you desire, such as good fortune or the clearing of negativity. Visualize the wind carrying your intentions far and wide. Alternatively, tie three knots in a piece of string or cord, with each knot representing a specific desire or intention. As you tie each knot, speak your request aloud to the wind. Once finished, release the string into the wind, allowing the air to carry your wishes.

Storm-Cutting Spell

(Europe)

This storm-cutting spell—using a blade to symbolically cut through a storm—is rooted mainly in European folk magic, especially Celtic, Norse, and Slavic traditions. Variations exist worldwide, but this simple act of cutting to redirect or disperse storm energy is a powerful, universal symbol. To perform a storm-cutting spell to ward off or dissipate a storm, take a sharp object, such as a knife or sword, and symbolically cut through the storm by directing the blade toward the sky or the direction the storm is coming from. While doing this, focus on the intention to dissipate or redirect the storm's energy. You may chant a prayer or incantation for protection, safety, or calm. The storm-cutting spell is a way to channel the forces of nature and bring balance or peace during turbulent weather.

Sun and Moon Water Charging

(Various Traditions)

Charging water with the energy of the sun or moon is a practice found across many folk magic traditions worldwide. In this practice, water is charged with the powerful energies of the sun or moon to enhance its magical properties. To charge water with sun energy, place a clear glass jar or bowl of water in direct sunlight for several hours, allowing it to absorb the sun's vitality, often for purposes like energizing spells or attracting abundance. For moon water, place the water under the light of the full moon, letting it soak in the lunar energy, which is often used for purification, emotional healing, or divination. Both practices harness celestial forces to empower the water for magical use in weather and nature magic, as well as other folk practices.

*　*　*

These traditional folk practices are found all over the world and are embraced by people from many different religions. That said, folk magic influenced by Catholicism and Christianity often seems more visible—although this may reflect a Western perspective, where these traditions are more obvious. There's also the way our awareness shapes what we notice. Once we recognize something, it appears everywhere. The spread of Christianity through missionaries and colonization certainly shaped many folk traditions, blending local customs with religious beliefs. I'm also interested in exploring how similar magical practices show up within other religions, to offer a broader comparison.

Jewish Folk Magic

Jewish folk magic is rooted in Kabbalah, Talmudic traditions, and regional folklore. Here are some common types of spells and rituals.

Protection and Warding Off Evil

- Amulet (*Kame'a*): This practice involves inscribing divine names or sacred verses—such as Psalm 91—onto parchment, metal, or other materials. These written amulets are used in Jewish folk magic to protect against illness, the evil eye, demons, and malevolent spirits.

- Red Thread Ritual: A red string often sourced from near Rachel's Tomb is wrapped around the wrist to guard against the *ayin hara*—the evil eye.

- Salt Circle: Sprinkling salt around a home or bed is a protective practice used to ward off harmful spirits, including *shedim* (malevolent spirits).

- Ketav Pitka (Protective or Petitionary): Also known as *ketav petek*, this is used to call in protection, healing, fertility, or divine help. Sacred names, Psalms, or prayers are written on a slip of paper or parchment and kept close—tucked into an amulet pouch, placed under a pillow, or even inserted into a crevice like the Western Wall. This practice is especially common in Kabbalistic, Sephardic, and Mizrahi Jewish traditions, but it also appears in Ashkenazi folk practice. It works like a written prayer or charm—meant to draw in spiritual aid.

- Hand of Miriam (Hamsa): This protective symbol is used in Jewish communities, especially among Sephardic and Mizrahi Jews, to ward off the evil eye and invite blessings. It shares regional roots with the Hand of Fatima and reflects a common tradition across Jewish and Muslim cultures in North Africa and the Middle East.

Love and Relationships

» Honey and Paper Spell: A beloved's name is written on paper, dipped in honey, and accompanied by a verse such as Song of Songs 6:3 ("I am my beloved's and my beloved is mine") to sweeten love or mend relationships. This folk charm draws on biblical symbolism and the spiritual power of words and sweetness.

» Rose Water Anointment: This practice involves anointing oneself or the home with rose water, sometimes infused with recited Psalms to draw in love, harmony, and spiritual grace. Common in Sephardic and Mizrahi traditions, it blends sacred text with sensory ritual.

Healing and Health

» Psalm Recitations: This practice involves chanting specific Psalms—like Psalm 30 for healing and recovery, or Psalm 121 for general protection—over those who are sick.

» Lead Pouring (*Bleigiessen*): In Central and Eastern Europe, lead pouring was part of the broader folk culture and was adopted by some Ashkenazi communities. This ritual involves pouring molten lead—or a safer alternative like tin—into water to diagnose the source of an illness or spiritual affliction, often related to the evil eye. The shapes formed in the water are then interpreted for insight and healing.

Prosperity and Good Fortune

» Bread and Salt Blessing: The practice of placing bread and salt at the entrance of a new home is a traditional blessing ritual symbolizing hospitality, protection, and abundance. It's meant to welcome guests and invite prosperity and good fortune into the household.

» Reciting Psalms: Reciting verses, like Psalm 23, is a common practice for protection and blessing. Sometimes this is combined with keeping symbolic items nearby—such as a silver coin under the pillow—to invite financial success and abundance.

Banishing and Exorcism

» Golem Creation is a practice in Jewish mystical traditions where a clay figure is animated through divine names to serve as a protector.

» *Ketav Pitka* (Written Expulsion) is the practice of driving something out. The name of an illness, malevolent spirit, curse, or negative force is written down on paper and cast into running water. By doing this, the practitioner sends the unwanted energy out of the body or space and back into the flow of nature. It's a ritual of release—meant to remove what does not belong. Many of these spells have been passed down orally and adapted over time, reflecting the rich regional diversity within Sephardic, Ashkenazi, and Mizrahi traditions.

Islamic Folk Magic

Often referred to in part by terms like Ruqyah (spiritual healing), Taweez (amulets), or Sihr (magic, sometimes considered forbidden), Islamic folk magic blends Quranic verses, traditional healing methods, and regional cultural practices. Across the Muslim world, many communities incorporate folk rituals for protection, healing, love, and prosperity—though views on these practices vary. Here are some commonly observed folk traditions.

Protection and Warding against Evil

- » Ruqyah (Spiritual Healing Recitations) involves reciting Quranic verses such as Surah Al-Falaq, Surah An-Nas, and Ayat al-Kursi over oneself or over water to protect against the evil eye, jinn, and malevolent magic.

- » Taweez (Amulets) are worn or carried for protection, typically containing Quranic verses, divine names, or prayers written on paper and enclosed in a locket or cloth pouch to ward off harm.

- » Burning incense such as frankincense is a common practice for purifying a space and driving away negative spirits, including jinn. The fragrant smoke is believed to cleanse the environment and create spiritual protection.

- » Hand of Fatima (Hamsa) Symbol is used in North African and Middle Eastern cultures to protect against the evil eye.

Love and Relationships

- » Rose Water and Sugar Spell is the practice of writing the names of two people on a piece of paper, placing it in rose water with sugar, and reciting verses like Surah Al-Fatiha to create harmony and love.

- » Seven Knots Spell is the practice of tying seven knots in a string while reciting Quranic verses to strengthen or mend relationships. The number seven is symbolically significant in many cultures and spiritual practices, including Islam.

Healing and Health

- » Honey and Black Seed Healing is the practice of mixing honey and black cumin seeds (*Nigella sativa*), both mentioned in Islamic tradition, with Surah Al-Fatiha recitations for physical and spiritual healing.

- » Drinking Ruqyah Water is the practice of drinking water over which Quranic verses have been recited. This traditional Islamic folk practice is used for healing physical illness and removing spiritual afflictions like jinn or the evil eye.

Prosperity and Good Fortune

- » Surah Al-Waqiah for Wealth is the practice of reciting Surah Al-Waqiah daily to attract financial stability and abundance. Many believe it brings blessings and prosperity when recited regularly.

- » Salt and Olive Oil Blessing is the practice of placing salt and olive oil at the entrance of a home while saying prayers for prosperity and protection.

Banishing and Exorcism

- » Ruqyah for Jinn Possession is performed by reciting Surah Al-Baqarah and Ayat al-Kursi over a possessed person or in a home to expel harmful spirits (jinn).

- » Seven Peppercorns Ritual is the practice of burning seven black peppercorns while reciting protective verses to remove curses or negative energy.

» Writing and Washing Spell is the practice of writing a protective verse on paper, dissolving it in water, and drinking it to remove spiritual blockages.

These practices shift and change depending on the region, blending influences from North Africa, the Middle East, South Asia, and Southeast Asia. Each culture shapes these rituals in its own way, keeping Islamic folk magic alive, vibrant, and deeply connected to local traditions.

Hindu Folk Magic

Hindu folk magic is a rich blend of Vedic teachings, Tantra, Ayurveda, and local traditions. It draws on mantras, yantras (sacred symbols), and rituals aimed at protection, love, healing, prosperity, and banishing negative forces. Here are some common spells and practices.

Protection and Warding Off Evil

» Lemon and Chili Totka is the practice of hanging a lemon and seven green chilies outside homes or businesses to ward off the evil eye.

» Black Thread Charm is the practice of tying a black thread around the wrist or ankle, often infused with mantras, to protect against negative energies.

» Kajal (Kohl) Protection is the practice of applying black kajal to a child's forehead or feet to shield them from the evil eye.

» Burning Camphor Ritual is the practice of waving burning camphor (kapur) around a person or space while reciting prayers to cleanse negativity.

Love and Relationships

- » Rose Petal and Saffron Spell is the practice of soaking rose petals in saffron-infused water while chanting the Kleem mantra to attract love.

- » Betel Leaf Ritual is the practice of writing the names of two lovers on a betel (*Piper betle*) leaf, wrapping it with red thread, and placing it under a pillow to strengthen relationships.

- » Shiva-Parvati Puja for Marriage is the practice of offering milk, honey, and flowers to a Shiva-Parvati idol while reciting prayers for a successful marriage.

Healing and Health

- » Tulsi (Holy Basil) Healing is the practice of boiling tulsi (*Ocimum sanctum*) leaves in water while chanting the Maha Mrityunjaya mantra for physical and spiritual healing.

- » Rudraksha Mala Therapy is the practice of wearing a rudraksha bead necklace, associated with Lord Shiva, for stress relief and energy balance.

- » Turmeric and Salt Bath is the practice of bathing in water mixed with turmeric and sea salt to cleanse illness and negative vibrations.

Prosperity and Good Fortune

- » Gomti Chakra Coin Ritual is the practice of keeping Gomti Chakra (sacred sea fossils) in a wallet or cash box for financial stability.

» Lighting Ghee Lamps on Thursdays is the practice of offering ghee lamps to Lord Vishnu or Goddess Lakshmi to attract wealth.

» Feeding Crows and Cows is the practice of offering food to crows (associated with honoring ancestors) and cows (sacred in Hinduism, symbolizing purity and abundance) for blessings and good karma.

Banishing and Exorcism

» Mustard Seed and Rock Salt Cleansing is the practice of tossing mustard seeds and rock salt into a fire while chanting mantras to dispel negative influences, break curses, and clear spiritual interference. This ritual is rooted in regional Hindu folk traditions for powerful energetic cleansing.

» Neem Leaf Smoke Ritual is the practice of burning dried neem (*Azadirachta indica*) leaves and wafting the smoke throughout the home to drive out evil spirits and cleanse the space. Neem has long been used in Hindu folk traditions for its purifying and protective properties.

» Lemon and Needle Curse Removal is the practice of piercing a lemon with needles and leaving it at a crossroads to draw out and dispel curses, hexes, or malevolent magic. The lemon is believed to absorb negativity, while the crossroads serves as a liminal space for release.

These practices vary widely across regions, shaped by local village customs, Ayurvedic principles, and Tantric influences, reflecting the deeply rooted and diverse nature of Hindu folk magic.

* * *

As you can see, folk magic is indeed a cultural practice, and folk practitioners across different cultures and religions share common practices.

These spells and rituals highlight the deep connection between culture, environment, and spirituality, showing how folk magic is a universal expression of human belief and tradition.

Curses and Countermeasures

Countermeasures include protections, shields, or actions taken to neutralize or block the effects of a curse or harmful magic. They are more about taking a proactive defense and remedying the situation.

1. The Evil Eye

(Mediterranean, Middle East, South Asia, Latin America, Eastern Europe)

How It's Done: The curse is believed to be cast through an envious or malicious gaze. No physical ritual is needed—just intense negative emotions directed at a person.

Some traditions enhance it by whispering a curse under the breath or using specific phrases.

Countermeasures: Wear a nazar (blue eye-shaped charm), hamsa, or red thread. Use an egg cleansing by rubbing an egg over the body and breaking it into water to diagnose the curse, to name a few different ones other than the typical Italian evil-eye cure.

2. Binding Spells

(Europe, African Diaspora)

How It's Done: Write the target's name on paper or cloth and tie it with black string or twine.

A poppet (doll) representing the person is wrapped in thread, buried, or placed in a jar of vinegar.

Knots in a rope or a "witch's ladder" (feathers tied into a braided cord) symbolize restriction.

Countermeasures: Unbind the knots, cut cords, or burn the paper with cleansing herbs like rosemary or rue.

3. Curse of the Jinni
(Middle East, North Africa, South Asia)

How It's Done: Write the person's name on a piece of paper and place it under a cursed object (like an old mirror or item taken from a graveyard). Or, invoke a jinni through fire, reciting a petition to harm the target. Another option is to bury a cursed talisman under their home or where they walk.

Countermeasures: Recite prayers like Ayat al-Kursi (Islamic tradition) or perform a smoke cleansing with frankincense. Destroy or purify the cursed object in running water.

4. The Bone-Pointing Curse
(Australia)

How It's Done: In some Indigenous Australian cultures, a shaman—often referred to as a kurdaitcha—carves and ritually empowers a bone, which is then pointed at a person as a curse. In some cases, the bone may be buried near the target's dwelling. The victim, believing deeply in the curse's power, may experience severe distress or even death.

Countermeasures: Healing and counter-rituals are performed by another traditional healer, who works to neutralize the curse's spiritual energy through song, ceremony, or other culturally specific practices.

5. The Footprint Curse

(Africa, India, Caribbean, Hoodoo Traditions of Southern United States)

How It's Done: This curse involves taking dirt from a person's footprint—believed to carry their essence—and mixing it with sulfur or graveyard dirt. The mixture is then placed back in their path or near their home to bring harm.

Countermeasures: Traditional protections include sweeping the ground after walking, washing shoes with salt water, or crossing a body of running water to break the spell's effect

6. The Pulled-Back Shadow Curse

(Southeast Asia, Philippines)

How It's Done: A practitioner steps on a person's shadow while calling their name backward or reciting an incantation. In extreme cases, a small part of the shadow is symbolically "cut" with a blade.

Countermeasures: Walk in moonlight or perform candlelight rituals to "reconnect" the shadow. This countermeasure needs to be performed by a healer.

7. The Mirror Curse

(China, Japan, Slavic Countries)

How It's Done: A mirror is used to trap a person's essence—by writing their name on it or capturing their reflection. Then it's smashed or buried to cause harm. In some Slavic and East Asian traditions, mirrors are believed to hold spiritual residue, making them potent tools for binding or cursing.

Countermeasures: To break the curse, mirror shards may be buried at a crossroads, purified with salt, or ritually cleansed with incantations or fire.

8. The Piss Bottle Curse

(European and Appalachian Folk Magic, Hoodoo)

How It's Done: The practitioner fills a bottle with their own urine, along with rusty nails, broken glass, and red pepper. The bottle is buried near the target's home to cause sickness or suffering.

Countermeasures: Dig up the bottle and break it under running water. Salt and herb cleansing rituals can also be used.

9. The Name Curse

(Europe, Asia, Africa, Caribbean, Americas)

The Name Curse shows up in folk traditions around the world—anywhere names are believed to hold spiritual power. You'll find versions of it in European magic (like Italian sorcery [*stregoneria*] and British cunning work), Hoodoo, Latin American brujería, South Asian and Jewish traditions, and across African and Afro-Caribbean practices where sympathetic name magic is common.

How It's Done: Write a person's name on paper and burn it while chanting their misfortune.

Some traditions carve the name on a candle and let it melt completely. This is based on the belief that harming the representation of a person (their name or image) can affect them directly.

Countermeasures: Burn a new name petition for healing and reversal. Some practices change the spelling of the afflicted person's name to break the curse.

* * *

I've only just scratched the surface of folk curses, but even this glimpse reveals something powerful: These aren't relics. They're still practiced today, often hand in hand with blessings, protections, and healing. Curses are part of the living current of folk magic—not separate from it, but woven right into its fabric. And in many ways, they're universal. Every culture has had its own way of righting injustice, redirecting harm, or restoring balance—especially when other systems fail. Folk curses speak to that ancient need to protect, to respond, and to hold power when there seems to be none.

Chapter 9

Conclusion

Folk magic is universal because it transcends both time and geography. People, regardless of culture, have always sought ways to influence their environment, protect themselves, and connect with unseen forces. This shared human desire to understand and control the world through magic, herbs, rituals, and spirituality is a thread that runs through every culture. While practices may differ in tools, rituals, and deities, the underlying beliefs about the power of nature, spirits, and personal agency are remarkably consistent across the world. Each culture adapts its practices based on its environment, available resources, and historical influences, making folk witchcraft both universal and wonderfully diverse.

Crafting Your Own Folk Magic Practice

Folk magic is more than just a set of practices; it's a worldview, a way of living that connects us to the natural world, the spirits of our ancestors, and the rhythms of the seasons. It's about seeing the magic in everyday life, finding meaning in the smallest moments, and embracing the interconnectedness of all things. Living this way means honoring tradition while making it personal, allowing ancient practices to evolve and blend into our modern lives. It's about using what is around you—local plants, the cycles of the moon, the energy of the land—to create something deeply meaningful, both spiritually and practically. In folk magic, magic isn't separate from life; it's a constant thread woven throughout our day-to-day existence.

A personal folk magic practice that honors your heritage and environment requires observation, research, and intuition. One of the most important aspects of a strong, evolving practice is the continuous flow between gathering knowledge and refining how you apply it. Rather than simply accumulating information, your focus should be on integrating what resonates with you, shaping a practice that feels both personal and effective.

Learning never truly stops—you'll return to reference books, seek out new perspectives, and refine your understanding over time. But this doesn't mean you have to hold on to every detail or rigidly follow every prescribed method. Instead, allow yourself the flexibility to engage with what feels relevant in the moment. Maybe you observe the moon phases closely for a while, then shift to a more intuitive approach. Perhaps you honor the seasonal cycles in a way that's meaningful to you, rather than following a strict ritual calendar.

Your practice should breathe, expand, and refine itself in a natural rhythm—always in motion, always deepening. Here's how to craft a practice deeply tied to natural cycles, cultural traditions, and local landscapes:

» **Observe the natural cycles:** Track the seasons, weather patterns, and moon phases where you live. Notice how plants, animals, and waterways change throughout the year. Align your spells and rituals with local agricultural cycles, such as planting, harvesting, or migration. For example, if you live near the ocean, incorporate tide magic into your practice. If in the mountains, work with stones, winds, and altitude-based plant medicine.

» **Research your cultural and ancestral traditions:** Explore folklore, magic, myths, and superstitions from your ancestors. Look into traditional seasonal festivals, healing methods, and spirit beliefs. If your ancestral roots are unclear, explore regional practices and other traditions that resonate with you.

» **Work with local spirits:** Learn about the magical properties of native plants. Connect with local spirits, land deities, or guardian ancestors. Use stones, shells, wood, or water from your environment in rituals and spell work.

» **Create a seasonal spiritual practice:** Celebrate solstices, equinoxes, and local harvest festivals. Make offerings to land spirits, ancestors, or natural forces. Develop personal rituals tied to seasonal shifts (such as a cleansing bath for spring or a bonfire for winter renewal).

» **Track changes and experiences:** Record seasonal shifts, successful spells, and any relevant folklore you discover. Note personal experiences with spirits, omens, and local energies.

» **Stay open:** Accept the possibility that spirits from other cultures may be connected to you. Perhaps they are distant ancestors reaching across time. Trust that what is meant for you will naturally find its way into your practice, while what isn't meant for you will remain beyond your grasp, no matter how much you seek it. Let this understanding guide you with both openness and discernment.

» **Embrace DIY:** Forage local materials and repurpose thrifted items into magical tools and objects. Craft your own incense, oils, poppets, and charm bags—infusing them with your energy and intent. This hands-on method deepens your connection to your craft and makes your practice uniquely yours.

Ultimately, your folk magic practice should feel personal, intuitive, and rooted in your ancestral and local culture. By aligning with nature and honoring cultural traditions, you create a spiritual and magical practice that is authentic, powerful, and deeply connected to who you are and where you live.

From Rue's Grimoire

I've always believed that magic is meant to be shared. What follows are some of my favorite incense blends, spells, and card meanings—pages pulled straight from my own grimoire. I offer them here with an open hand, so you can tuck them into your own magical book if they speak to you. Take what resonates, adapt what you need, and let your practice grow.

> **Warning:** Do not handle, create, or use any of these recipes if you are pregnant, breastfeeding, or suspect that you may be pregnant. Always exercise caution when working with herbs, oils, and incense. It is recommended to perform a patch test before using any new ingredients on your skin. Keep all products away from children and pets.

Rue's Nay-Pahm Incense Blend (Used to Banish Evil Spirits)

I blend my love of loose incense with the plants and resins my ancestors used in their healing and magic. Following ancient traditions, I create a versatile coarse powder for cleansing spaces by fumigation against disease and negative energies. I make it during the full moon and, more recently, have used a Vitamix for a finer blend (optional). The sharp blades add an extra edge—pun intended! If you choose this method, I strongly recommend wearing safety goggles and a face mask.

Ingredients (all dried herbs)

4 parts mugwort (*Artemisia vulgaris*)

1 part snakeroot (*Bistorta officinalis*)

1 part spikenard (*Nardostachys jatamansi*)

1 part wormwood (*Artemisia absinthium*)

1 part agrimony (*Agrimonia eupatoria*)

1 part hyssop (*Hyssopus officinalis*)

1 part dogwood (*Cornus florida*)

½ part rosemary (*Salvia rosmarinus*) leaves

1 part coarsely ground cloves (*Syzygium aromaticum*)

Store in an airtight glass jar. Leave it to charge at least until the next full moon.

I cannot stress this enough: You only need to use a tiny bit—¼ teaspoon to ½ teaspoon.

I toast the blend in an herb burner or oil warmer lined with tin foil, but never leave it unattended as it can self-ignite and start a fire. When heavy energies need clearing, it will smoke and ignite; when it toasts gently, less clearing is needed. It primarily smells like cloves. Ensure the room is well-ventilated and keep it away from children and pets.

I save the charred remains in a small cast-iron cauldron to make black salt. I use this blend to cleanse my home of negative energies and spirits, especially during cold and flu season. A little goes a long way, and I typically use it only a few times a year.

This blend is versatile: For oil, mix it with resins; for other incense types, add it to small glass pendants and amulets, and use it to dress candles.

Rue's Chthonic Mother Oil

(Inspired by Her scent when I invoke Her. This is the closest I have come to replicating what I smell when She is present.)

Ingredients

2 nuggets styrax (*Styrax benzoin*) resin

1 nugget myrrh (*Commiphora myrrha*) resin

22.5 ml patchouli (*Pogostemon cablin*) essential oil

6 drops cypress (*Cupressus sempervirens*) essential oil

6 drops benzoin (*Styrax benzoin*) essential oil

3 drops birch tar (*Betula pendula*) essential oil

In a mortar and pestle, grind the resins to a fine powder. I pour everything into a brown glass bottle with a secure lid. I give it all a firm shake and store it in a dark cupboard to do its thing for about three months. I give the bottle a firm shake once a week for the first month and then at least every two to three weeks afterward. My last batch took over six months to finally smell blended and smooth, so be patient.

Rue's Queen of Heaven Oil

Ingredients

2 parts rose fragrance oil

1 part African musk fragrance oil

Dried rose petals

I use the fragrance oils sold at metaphysical shops: 20 ml of rose fragrance oil and 10 ml African musk fragrance oil. Sometimes I bump up the musk, depending on how I'm feeling. I pour it all in a brown glass bottle large enough to fit the oils and a teaspoon or two of rose petals. Give it a good shake and leave it alone in the dark for three months.

Rue's Naples Water

This recipe is inspired by the flavors used in the Neapolitan Easter pie. A wonderful offering to the souls of the dead any time of year.

Ingredients

- 2 bottles of orange flower water (food grade, typically found in the ethnic aisle of supermarkets; you can always use more)
- 1 large cinnamon stick
- Zest of one whole orange (I wash the orange first and use a vegetable peeler to shave off just the zest and avoid the pith)
- Zest of one whole lemon (same as I did with the orange)

I place everything in a pot and heat it up to just before boiling. Transfer everything to a clean glass jar that is airtight and leave it to cool on the kitchen counter overnight. It's ready to use the next day. I remove the orange and lemon zest; then I pour some of the water into a bowl and leave it out as an offering to the souls of the dead and as a room spray.

Onion Love Spell

My very first spell-casting experience.

Ingredients

- 1 onion (yellow or red onion)
- 6 pins or nails
- A quiet space, with an open closet or drawer

1. Hold the onion in your hands and think deeply about the person you wish to connect with or the type of love bond you wish to create. Focus on the idea of shared connection and the concept that love often manifests in physical and emotional forms.

2. Stick the pins or nails into the onion while concentrating on your intention of forming a love bond. As you pin the onion, think of how this bond will grow and be sealed through shared experiences (symbolized by the cuts).

3. Stand with your back to an open closet or a hidden space. This symbolizes the secrets of the relationship and the magical workings that are still unfolding.

4. Throw the onion over your shoulder into the closet or hidden space. As you do this, envision the two of you eventually crossing paths and beginning your relationship. The onion's pins represent the connection between you.

5. The next time you meet the person you wish to form a connection with (or already know), when you both accidentally sustain cuts on your hands, the person with the largest cut is believed to love the other more. This physical injury is a symbol of emotional vulnerability and the unequal but deeply connected love that will grow between you.

6. Leave the onion undisturbed in the closet or hidden space, allowing the magic to unfold naturally as time passes.

Symbolism

Onion: Represents layers of connection and the growth of love.

Pins: Bind the intention and the bond.

Number 6: Symbolizes love.

Closet/hidden space: Symbolizes the unseen forces at work, protecting the relationship's privacy until the right moment.

Cuts: A physical manifestation of emotional bonding and vulnerability. The person with the largest cut is thought to love the other more—a symbolic "mark" of affection.

This spell plays with the idea of sympathetic magic, where the physical injury (in the form of cuts) serves as a sign of the emotional dynamics between two people. It's both a binding spell and a test of love.

Cartomancy for Fortune-Telling and Spell Work

Cartomancy has deep roots in various traditions of fortune-telling with playing cards. The meanings of the suits, court cards, and numbers have been shaped by centuries of practice and interpretation. What follows is a synthesis of commonly accepted meanings in cartomancy, reflecting how readers have worked with the standard fifty-two-card deck over time.

Suits

Hearts (♥): Emotions, Relationships, and Matters of the Heart

Represents love, emotions, relationships, family, and connections.
Focuses on matters of the heart, emotional fulfillment, and personal connections.

Diamonds (♦): Material Wealth, Career, and Success

Represents financial matters, career, business, material possessions, and success.
Concerns goals, achievements, and physical aspects of life, including wealth and resources.

Clubs (♣): Action, Work, and Challenges

Represents energy, work, action, challenges, and growth.
Often linked to effort, progress, and overcoming obstacles.

Spades (♠): Intellect, Conflict, and Transformation

Represents thoughts, communication, challenges, conflicts, and transformation.
Associated with mental energy, decision-making, and transitions in life.

Court Cards

Court cards represent different types of people or personalities and often give insight into individuals or influences in a reading.

Jack:

Represents messages, young or immature energy, curiosity, or someone who is learning.

In some cases, the Jack can indicate a person who is inexperienced or naive.

Knight:

Represents movement, action, and courage.

Often symbolizes someone who is pursuing goals, embarking on a journey, or is active in their life.

Queen:

Represents nurturing, intuition, and maturity.

Often symbolizes a strong, supportive woman or someone who embodies qualities of emotional intelligence and care.

King:

Represents authority, leadership, and wisdom.

Symbolizes a powerful, confident individual or someone in a position of power and control.

Numbers

Ace:

Represents new beginnings, opportunities, and potential.
Signifies a fresh start, an invitation, or an initiation.

Two:

Represents balance, partnerships, and duality.

Focuses on relationships, choices, or decisions that involve two elements.

Three:

Represents growth, expansion, and creativity.

Often indicates cooperation, teamwork, or the emergence of something new.

Four:

Represents stability, structure, and foundation.

Focuses on solidifying plans, creating security, or building long-term success.

Five:

Represents change, conflict, and challenge.

Signals a time of tension, struggle, or the need to adapt to shifting circumstances.

Six:

Represents harmony, balance, and adjustment.

Signifies the resolution of conflicts, a return to harmony, or a period of peace.

Seven:

Represents reflection, introspection, and spiritual growth.

Often indicates a moment of pause, contemplation, or spiritual insight.

Eight:

Represents power, achievement, and material success.

Focuses on ambition, progress, and reaching a goal.

Nine:

Represents completion, fulfillment, and wisdom.

Often signifies the nearing of an ending, the conclusion of a cycle, or a period of reflection and realization.

Ten:

Represents culmination, fulfillment, and transformation.

Often symbolizes the end of a cycle, completion, or the final stages of a journey.

Combinations and Contextual Meanings

In cartomancy, meaning doesn't live in just one card; it unfolds in the relationships between them. The combination of cards, their proximity, and the order in which they appear can shift the tone of a reading entirely. For instance, the Ace of Hearts might point to a fresh emotional bond or heartfelt offering, but if it's followed by the Ten of Diamonds, the message could deepen into something about a prosperous union or emotional fulfillment linked to financial stability.

Context is everything. A card's meaning can brighten or darken depending on what surrounds it. A Queen may be nurturing in one spread and scheming in another, depending on who sits beside her. That's why paying close attention to pairings, clusters, and positions in a spread is vital. This layered language of symbols allows for nuanced, grounded readings—ones that truly reflect the complexities of life. Learning to read these patterns is like hearing the cards speak in full sentences rather than single words.

Cartomancy follows a formula and interpreting the cards is an art. Each practitioner develops their own rhythm, spreads, and way of placing the cards over time. I recommend starting with a simple three-card spread—reading from left to right—to get a feel for the meanings, the directionality, and how the cards begin to speak to one another.

There are plenty of cartomancy resources out there—books, videos, and guides—and I encourage you to explore what resonates with you. But at the end of the day, we truly learn by doing, by laying down the cards and letting them speak.

Just as I opened this section with an open hand, I'll close it the same way. These spells, blends, and card meanings are living pieces of my practice, and now they're yours to shape. May they inspire, guide, and root you in your own path—because magic grows best when it's tended with care and shared in good spirit.

Chapter 10

Unearthing the Roots
A Practical Guide to Finding Information

Folk magic is deeply intertwined with every aspect of life, and its influence can be found in a wide range of areas. It's not limited to sources specifically focused on magic itself; rather, it is present in many cultural practices and beliefs. To uncover a wealth of information about folk magic, we can look beyond traditional texts on magic and explore resources related to low magic, practical magic, mysticism, and folk religion. Folk customs, herbalism, cultural history, anthropology, and even mythology all hold valuable insights into the practices and symbols that shape folk magic. Additionally, folklore, fairy tales, and classic literature often contain hidden references and magical elements that reflect the influence of folk magic in everyday life. In essence, folk magic is not just a practice, but also a lens through which we can better understand the interconnectedness of culture, spirituality, and the natural world.

To learn about local folk magic customs, you can gather valuable information from several places. Local tourist information centers often provide insights into regional traditions and folklore, while city halls and museums may offer historical context and displays related to local customs. Libraries are excellent resources for books and research on the subject, and they provide access to archival material. Heritage sites, which preserve the cultural history of a region, can offer a direct connection to ancient practices. Farmers' markets are another great resource, where local sellers may share herbal remedies, charms, and folk traditions passed down through generations. Ethnic grocery stores, especially those catering to specific cultural communities, may carry items related to folk magic, such as herbs, candles, and talismans, and can be a gateway to learning about the magical practices tied to particular cultures. These places collectively offer a rich tapestry of local knowledge about folk magic customs, often directly rooted in the region's cultural heritage.

> Note: One of the best ways to access the most accurate and authentic information about cultural folk magic is by consulting sources written in the language of the specific culture you're researching. Many traditional practices, beliefs, and rituals are deeply rooted in the language and worldview of the community, and translated materials can sometimes lose important nuances. Learning the language of your ancestors holds immense value when practicing their folk magic: It allows you to connect more deeply with their cultural expressions, rituals, and spiritual practices, preserving the authenticity of the traditions. Fortunately, we live in an amazing time where technology makes it easier than ever to access these original sources. Translator applications and online language courses offer valuable tools to help you understand materials in foreign languages. When doing online research, try searching for terms such as *folk customs*, *folk religion*, *folk medicine*, *superstitious beliefs*, *folklore*, *cultural holidays*, and *syncretism* in the language of the culture you're studying. This approach can lead you to a richer and more authentic understanding of folk magic traditions and a deeper personal connection to your ancestral practices.

Living Folk Magic is the culmination of my personal experiences and my journey of learning and comparing customs from people of different cultures and religions. It has been incredibly enriching. Through personal conversations, I've gained unique insights into rituals, herbs, and beliefs that aren't always found in books or academic sources. It's fascinating to hear firsthand accounts of practices passed down through generations, from protective charms to complex spiritual rituals. Attending cultural events, festivals, and religious gatherings, as well as connecting with like-minded individuals in metaphysical shops or online communities, including social media platforms, has helped me uncover a wealth of knowledge. Online spaces such as Facebook groups, Reddit threads, and YouTube have been particularly valuable. On YouTube, I've found long-form content where both learning and seasoned practitioners share their experiences and insightful wisdom, offering in-depth tutorials, stories, and discussions on various folk magic practices. These resources have allowed me to engage directly with knowledgeable individuals from diverse backgrounds, enhancing my understanding of folk magic. Engaging with others who share similar interests has not only deepened my knowledge but also provided a greater appreciation for the diversity and depth of global spiritual practices. These experiences, both in person and online, have been invaluable in shaping the content of this book, allowing me to bring a personal and authentic perspective to the subject.

Here are some resources to get you started.

Books

Norse and Scandinavian Folk Magic

1. *Icelandic Folk Magic: Witchcraft of the North* by Albert Björn Shiell
   ISBN: 978-1959883289
   Description: A guide to the ancient and modern traditions of Icelandic folk magic, including runes, charms, and spells used for healing and protection.

2. *Northern Mysteries & Magick: Runes & Feminine Powers* by Freya Aswynn
ISBN: 978-1567180473
Description: A book on Norse runes and their spiritual significance, emphasizing the feminine aspects of Norse magic and their connection to the divine.

3. *Trolldom: Spells and Methods of the Norse Folk Magic Tradition* by Johannes Björn Gårdbäck
ISBN: 978-0990313618
Description: A deep dive into the practical aspects of Norse magic, focusing on the methods, spells, and rituals used by ancient and modern practitioners.

Folk Magic in European, Middle Eastern, and Slavic Traditions

1. *The Ancestral Power of Amulets, Talismans, and Mascots* by Nigel Pennick
ISBN: 978-1644112205
Description: A guide to the history, uses, and significance of amulets, talismans, and mascots in folk magic and various religious traditions.

2. *The Cunning Man's Handbook* by Jim Baker
ISBN: 978-1905297689
Description: A practical guide to the craft of the cunning man, covering spells, charms, divination, and healing techniques rooted in folk magic.

3. *The Encyclopedia of Jewish Myth, Magic & Mysticism* by Geoffrey W. Dennis
ISBN: 978-0738745916
Description: A comprehensive reference on Jewish mysticism, magic, and mythology, exploring the key figures, rituals, and practices in Jewish magical traditions.

4. *The Evil Eye* by Antonio Pagliarulo
ISBN: 978-1578637973
Description: A comprehensive guide to the belief in the evil

eye across different cultures. The book explores the history, symbolism, and rituals associated with the evil eye, and includes practical advice on protection and warding off its harmful effects.

5. *Italian Folk Magic: Rue's Kitchen Witchery* by Mary-Grace Fahrun
   ISBN: 978-1578636181
   Description: A practical guide to Italian folk magic, including spells, rituals, and kitchen witchery that draws on ancient traditions and family wisdom.

6. *Jewish Magic and Superstition: A Study in Folk Religion* by Joshua Trachtenberg
   ISBN: 978-1614274070
   Description: An in-depth study of Jewish magical and superstitious practices, examining the intersection of religion, folklore, and magic in Jewish communities.

7. *Slavic Witchcraft: Old World Conjuring Spells and Folklore* by Natasha Helvin
   ISBN: 978-1620558423
   Description: A look into the magical practices and folklore of Eastern Europe, with a focus on Slavic traditions, rituals, and spells for protection and healing.

Spiritual and Folk Traditions in the Americas

1. *Animal-Wise* by Ted Andrews
   ISBN: 978-1888767636
   Description: A guide to understanding the symbolic meanings of animals in folklore, mythology, and spiritual traditions. The book explores the traits and wisdom associated with different animals and how they can be used as totems or guides in personal spiritual practices.

2. *Backwoods Witchcraft: Conjure & Folk Magic from Appalachia* by Jake Richards

ISBN: 978-1578636532
Description: A collection of Appalachian folk magic traditions, including conjure spells, healing practices, and the mystical arts passed down through generations.

3. *A Deck of Spells: Hoodoo Playing Card Magic in Rootwork and Conjure* by Charles Porterfield
ISBN: 978-0971961289
Description: A collection that offers readers over one hundred spells, charms, and authentic old-time divination methods, illustrating how playing cards have been employed for both fortune-telling and magical work.

4. *Mexican Sorcery: A Practical Guide to Brujería de Rancho* by Laura Davila
ISBN: 978-1578637812
Description: A practical guide to Mexican folk magic, focusing on Brujería, spells, and rituals rooted in Indigenous and colonial traditions.

5. *Power of the Psalms* by Anna Riva
ISBN: 978-1943138609
Description: A spiritual guide that explores the use of the biblical Psalms for various aspects of daily life, including work, health, love, and success.

6. *Sister Karol's Book of Spells, Blessings & Folk Magic* by Karol Jackowski
ISBN: 978-1578636457
Description: A collection of simple spells, blessings, and folk magic rituals, with practical advice for using magic in everyday life.

7. *Sticks, Stones, Roots, and Bones* by Stephanie Rose Bird
ISBN: 978-0738702759
Description: A comprehensive guide to African American folk magic, herbology, and spirituality, drawing from African, Native American, and European traditions.

Herbs, Incense, and Magical Plants

1. *Ashkenazi Herbalism: Rediscovering the Herbal Traditions of Eastern European Jews* by Deatra Cohen and Adam Siegel
   ISBN: 978-1623175443
   Description: A detailed exploration of herbal traditions in Eastern European Jewish culture, blending folk medicine with spiritual practices.

2. *The Complete Book of Incense, Oils, and Brews* by Scott Cunningham
   ISBN: 978-0875421285
   Description: A detailed guide to creating your own magical oils, incense, and brews, offering recipes for spiritual and ritual use.

3. *Cunningham's Encyclopedia of Magical Herbs* by Scott Cunningham
   ISBN: 978-0875421223
   Description: An essential guide to the magical properties of herbs, their uses in rituals, spells, and healing practices across various spiritual traditions.

4. *Icelandic Plant Magic* by Albert Björn Shiell
   ISBN: 978-1959883111
   Description: A study of plants and herbs used in Icelandic folk magic traditions, with practical instructions on how to use these plants for magical purposes.

5. *The Witching Herbs: 13 Essential Plants and Herbs for Your Magical Garden* by Harold Roth
   ISBN: 978-1578635993
   Description: A guide to thirteen key magical herbs, their uses in witchcraft, and how to cultivate them for spiritual and ritual work.

Animism and Spirit World

1. *Aboriginal Men of High Degree: Initiation and Sorcery in the World's Oldest Tradition* by A. P. Elkin
   ISBN: 978-0892814213
   Description: An exploration of the secret initiation rites, spiritual beliefs, and shamanic practices of Aboriginal Australian elders.

2. *Animism: Respecting the Living World* by Graham Harvey
   ISBN: 978-0231137010
   Description: An exploration of animism, the belief that all life, including nonhuman entities, possesses a spirit or soul, and its significance in modern spiritual practices.

3. *Becoming Animal: An Earthly Cosmology* by David Abram
   ISBN: 978-0375713699
   Description: A philosophical work that discusses the connection between humans and animals, nature, and the cosmos, emphasizing animistic perspectives.

3. *Cunning Folk and Familiar Spirits: Shamanistic Visionary Traditions in Early Modern British Witchcraft and Magic* by Emma Wilby
   ISBN: 978-1845190798
   Description: A scholarly examination of the role of cunning folk and their familiar spirits in early modern British witchcraft, blending history and folklore.

4. *Engaging the Spirit World* edited by Lupa
   ISBN: 978-1905713325
   Description: A collection of essays about interacting with spirits and the spirit world, exploring shamanism, spirit work, and animism in contemporary practices.

5. *The Handbook of Contemporary Animism* edited by Graham Harvey
   ISBN: 978-1138928978
   Description: A collection of essays exploring contemporary animism, its practices, and its role in modern spirituality.

Spiritual and Folk Traditions in Asia

1. *Chinese Witchcraft* by Joseph Needham
   ISBN: 978-0710607952
   Description: A study of Chinese magical practices, including astrology, Taoism, alchemy, and spirit communication.

2. *The Magic of India* by Ajit Prakashan
   ISBN: 978-8180562542
   Description: A comprehensive guide to Indian folk magic, including mantras, talismans, astrology, and spiritual healing rooted in Hinduism and Tantra.

Magical Texts, Grimoires, and Encyclopedias

1. *Encyclopedia of Mystics, Saints, and Sages* by Judika Illes
   ISBN: 978-0062009579
   Description: This work offers biographies and insights into the lives and teachings of mystics, saints, and sages from around the world. It includes figures from different religious traditions and focuses on their spiritual practices and contributions to mystical thought.

2. *Encyclopedia of Spirits* by Judika Illes
   ISBN: 978-0061350245
   Description: This encyclopedia is a vast reference work that details over one thousand spirits, deities, and supernatural beings from various cultures and traditions. It offers historical context, rituals, and the lore surrounding each entity, making it an invaluable resource for practitioners of magic and spirituality.

3. *The Golden Bough: A Study in Magic and Religion* by Sir James George Frazer
   ISBN: 978-1645940210
   Description: A foundational work examining the connections

between religion, magic, and mythology across cultures, with a focus on rituals and sacrificial rites.

4. *The Night Battles: Witchcraft and Agrarian Cults in the Sixteenth and Seventeenth Centuries* by Carlo Ginzburg
ISBN: 978-1421409924
Description: An exploration of rural Italian witchcraft and agrarian cults, focusing on the social and magical practices of peasants in early modern Europe.

5. *The Sun of Knowledge (Shams al-Ma'arif)* by Ahmad Ibn 'Ali Al-Buni
ISBN: 978-1947544352
Description: A significant Arabic grimoire offering spells and invocations for various purposes, with a focus on spiritual growth, protection, and empowerment.

Acknowledgments

To everyone at Weiser Books—thank you for being phenomenal partners in this process. Your dedication, professionalism, and support have made this book possible. I'm honored to be part of your publishing family.

To my editor, Judika Illes—my mentor, literary midwife, and dear friend. I am forever grateful for your insight, guidance, and patience. Your belief in me has shaped every step of this work.

To my copy editor, Chuck Hutchinson—thank you for your work previously on *Italian Folk Magic* and now on *Living Folk Magic*. I'm deeply grateful for your attention to detail and your gift for organizing my thoughts in a way that reflects my vision with such care and clarity.

To my husband, Ray—your fierce love sustains me. You've grounded me through every part of this journey. Thank you for believing in me, especially in the moments when I couldn't believe in myself.

To my children, Brenna, Brigid, and Brigid's partner, Robin—thank you for your unconditional love and for being my light. I'm endlessly proud of each of you. You are already doing great things, and the best is yet to come.

To Laurie Fox—my dear friend, thank you for your unconditional love, your wisdom, and for always showing up with your heart wide open.

To Emile Vidmar—your generous and open heart, creative spirit, artistic talent, and capacity for reinvention are a constant inspiration.

To Sylvain Dubé—your guidance, encouragement, and steady belief in me have meant more than words can say. Thank you for being my friend.

To Nancy Shellito—thank you for your friendship and steady support over the years, and for generously sharing your magical craft with me.

To Ian Bernardo—you're a mensch.

To Hilarie Burton Morgan—thank you for championing my first book, *Italian Folk Magic*. Your continued support has meant the world to me.

To my Patreon members, Instagram followers, YouTube subscribers, and the vibrant community in Rue's Kitchen Facebook Group—thank you for your enthusiasm, encouragement, and the radiant energy you bring to our shared space. You inspire me every day and are an integral part of this journey.

Finally, to everyone who helped bring this book into being—whether named here or not—thank you for sharing your cultural folk practices and your wisdom. I carry your support with deep gratitude.

About the Author

Mary-Grace Fahrun was born in Bridgeport, Connecticut, to Italian immigrant parents and grew up in the Italian neighborhoods of Connecticut and Montreal. She is the author of the influential book *Italian Folk Magic: Rue's Kitchen Witchery* and the creatrix of Rue's Kitchen, her website dedicated to the preservation of Italian folk practices. Mary-Grace resides in British Columbia, Canada. Visit her at *rueskitchen.com*, on Instagram @rueskitchen, and on YouTube @MaryGraceFahrun.

To Our Readers

Weiser Books, an imprint of Red Wheel/Weiser, publishes books across the entire spectrum of occult, esoteric, speculative, and New Age subjects. Our mission is to publish quality books that will make a difference in people's lives without advocating any one particular path or field of study. We value the integrity, originality, and depth of knowledge of our authors.

Our readers are our most important resource, and we appreciate your input, suggestions, and ideas about what you would like to see published.

Visit our website at *www.redwheelweiser.com*, where you can learn about our upcoming books and free downloads, and also find links to sign up for our newsletter and exclusive offers.

You can also contact us at *info@rwwbooks.com* or at

Red Wheel/Weiser, LLC
65 Parker Street, Suite 7
Newburyport, MA 01950